Social Work Practice in Health Care

Social Work Practice in Health Care

EDITED BY

Mieke Badawi and Brenda Biamonti

WOODHEAD–FAULKNER

NEW YORK LONDON TORONTO SYDNEY TOKYO SINGAPORE

Published by Woodhead–Faulkner Limited,
Simon & Schuster International Group,
Fitzwilliam House, 32 Trumpington Street,
Cambridge CB2 1QY, England

First published 1990

© Woodhead–Faulkner Limited, 1990

British Library Cataloguing in Publication Data

Social work practice in health care.
1. Great Britain. Health services. Welfare work
I. Badawi, Mieke II. Biamonti, Brenda
362.10425

ISBN 0–85941–654–2

Library of Congress Cataloging in Publication Data

Designed by Geoff Green
Typeset by Quorn Selective Repro Ltd., Loughborough, Leicestershire
Printed in Great Britain by BPCC Wheatons Ltd, Exeter

It is much more important to know what sort of patient has a disease than to know what sort of disease a patient has.

C. H. Parry (1755–1822)

Contents

Preface

The implementation of the White Paper, *Caring for People*, will mean changes in the management and practice of social work, particularly at the interface between area health authorities and social services departments.

Social work in hospitals has a long and proud tradition. Its practitioners have always played an important part in ensuring that more than physical needs are met and have seen themselves as providing a bridge between the hospital and the community.

In the future, a duty laid on the local authority to 'assess individuals' needs in collaboration with medical, nursing and other agencies', will mean that their role will be even more crucial to ensure that the social and emotional needs of sick, disabled, frail and dying people continue to be met.

This book is an introduction to social work in a health setting, written by practitioners to answer the recurring question: But what do you actually do? There are very few texts that we can advise the enquirer to read and we felt it was time this gap was filled, particularly at this time of change in both health and social services. We hope this book will be read by other social work colleagues, who will in the future need to work even more closely with hospital and other NHS personnel, our colleagues in the health professions, who in their turn will have to collaborate more with social services personnel, social work and other students, and interested laymen.

The editors felt that the use of him/her in the text would be clumsy and therefore decided – on the toss of a coin – that 'she' would be used throughout the book where the gender of the subject could be either. We have aimed at using 'social worker' throughout, but in some contexts the use of 'hospital social worker', or the now somewhat old-fashioned sounding term 'medical social worker' was unavoidable. Similarly the person seeking help at the hospital is sometimes referred to as 'client', sometimes as 'patient'. In some contexts 'patient' seemed to be the correct term to use.

All of us working in the social and health services care for people and we shall have to do this *together* more than ever before. We hope this book will help us towards greater mutual understanding to the benefit of all clients/patients.

MIEKE BADAWI
BRENDA BIAMONTI
Oxford, spring 1990

Contributors

JULIET AUER, CQSW, MPhil (Southampton): Trained in Ericksonian Psychotherapy, and Psycho-Sexual Counselling. European Editor of American Association of Nephrology Social Work Journal. At present Social Worker to Oxford Regional Renal Unit.

MIEKE BADAWI, Diploma of Social Work (generic) from the Amsterdam Academy of Social work, AIMSW: Taught at the Higher Institute of Social Service, Alexandria, Egypt for six years. Extensive experience of Medical Social Work in this country. Until recently Senior Social Worker at the Nuffield Orthopaedic Centre, Oxford.

BRENDA BIAMONTI, CQSW, MSc (Leeds): Seventeen years experience of social work in a range of settings. Practising Gestalt Psychotherapist. Unit Manager (Disability), Northamptonshire Social Services.

JEAN CARR, BSc, CQSW, DipSW: Accredited member of the British Association of Psychotherapy. Has experience in health and community settings. At present Divisional Director (Health), Oxfordshire Social Services Department.

MARDI CHANDLER, MA (Medical Social Work, Chicago), MA TCD: Many years of hospital social work experience in this country. At present Head Social Worker, John Radcliffe I Hospital, Oxford.

ROSEMARY CLARIDGE, MA (Edin.), MSc (London): Has worked in child guidance and has extensive experience as a paediatric social worker in hospital. At present Senior Social Worker, John Radcliffe Hospital, Oxford.

MARGARET COPPEARD, CQSW: Sixteen years experience in both field and hospital settings, mainly in East London. Three years Principal Social Worker Harold Wood Hospital. At present Care Manager (Elderly), London Borough of Havering.

JENNY LEE, CQSW: Extensive experience in social work. At present Senior Social Worker, Nuffield Orthopaedic Centre, Oxford.

NIGEL PARSONS, BA CQSW: Nine years experience as social worker in inner London area team. Six years hospital experience. At present Principal Officer (General Hospitals) Oxfordshire County Council.

MARGARET ROSS, MA (Edin.), Diploma in Social Study, CQSW: At present Social Worker, John Radcliffe Hospital, Oxford.

ANABEL SHELLEY, CQSW (Ruskin, Oxford), MA (Brunel): At present Social Worker, Hugh Ellis Paediatric Assessment Centre, Churchill Hospital, Oxford.

SYLVIA STEVENSON, Certificate in Social Study (Edin.), AIMSW: At present Head Social Worker, John Radcliffe II Hospital, Oxford.

CHRISTINE TULLOCH, BA Social Administration (Nottingham), AIMSW: At present Social Worker, John Radcliffe Hospital, Oxford.

JUDITH UNWIN, MA, AIMSW: Many years experience as Hospital Social Worker in the United Kingdom and Australia. At present Senior Social Worker, John Radcliffe Hospital, Oxford.

CHAPTER 1

Historical perspectives

MIEKE BADAWI

Social workers in hospitals have sometimes felt that their role and *raison d'etre* have been misunderstood. Looking at their history it is interesting to see how often the same problems crop up in descriptions and discussions about hospital social work through the decades. There are three recurring themes: (a) the difference in perception of the task of the social worker between the workers themselves and the management and staff of the institution they work in; (b) the relationship between the medical and the social work professions; and (c) the fact that hospital social workers see a need for their special skills outside the hospitals, e.g. in general medical practices, a need which is not felt by that outside world – or not much. The seeds for these difficulties were sown quite early on in the life of the hospital social workers, or the almoners, as they were known (the prefix 'lady' was in fact exclusive to St Thomas' Hospital, London, the executive board of which had from its earliest days included six 'almoners', and the new almoner–social worker had to be called something slightly different.)

1.1 HISTORY 1885–1974

1.1.1 1885–1920

As charitable institutions hospitals were always short of money, and obliged to justify to donors the way their gifts were spent. By the end of the last century there was great anxiety lest people who could pay for treatment received free medical relief at the hospitals. However, social workers like Sir Charles Loch

1

of the Charity Organisation Society (COS, now the Family Welfare Association – FWA) had slightly different concerns: he pointed out in 1885 that there was a need in hospitals for a 'charitable assessor, or co-ordinator . . . well instructed as to all forms of relief other than medical . . . . His office should be to supplement the work of the medical officer by obtaining the general assistance without which medical relief will often fail in its purpose.'[1] He proposed in 1891 to a committee of the House of Lords, that 'trained social workers should be appointed to hospitals to determine the need of those who applied for medical relief', and in 1892 he wrote: 'At the present time, what more glaring picture of charitable impotence is there than that destitute persons should constantly apply to a free dispensary for drugs which cannot benefit them if they lack the necessary food.' In 1894 the Charity Organisation Society approached the board of the Royal Free Hospital with the offer of a trained worker for an experimental period and the first almoner, Miss Mary Stewart, was appointed to the Royal Free in 1895, her salary being paid conjointly by the Hospital and the COS.

The hospital board saw her duties as follows:
1. To prevent abuse of the hospital by persons able to pay for medical treatment.
2. To refer patients already in receipt of parish relief, and such as are destitute, to the Poor Law authorities.
3. To recommend suitable persons to join provident dispensaries.[2]

Sir Charles Loch saw her duties as follows:
1. To check the abuse of the out-patient department by patients who are either in a position to pay for treatment, or too poor to benefit by any treatment or assistance other than that obtainable through the Poor Law.
2. To ensure as far as possible that all patients to whom treatment has been granted should benefit to the full by that treatment.

It is clear that the board had a different perception of the almoner's duties from Sir Charles: the former was anxious to reduce the demands upon the hospital, the latter was more concerned with the needs of the patients. Miss Stewart seems to have been able to reconcile the two: she obviously gained the trust and respect of the hospital board, witness the fact that she remained at the hospital for many years, and her colleagues spoke of her with great respect for her qualities as a social worker. In the following ten years seven other hospital boards appointed their own almoners. They had all been trained by the COS and saw themselves as social workers first and foremost, with the patient's welfare at the centre of their work, which, as we have already noted, was not always the way the hospital board viewed their duties. Most of them were women of independent mind and character, and seem to have been able to make their presence felt and accepted in the hospitals, gradually introducing more of the kind of work they wanted to do and less of what the hospital expected of them.

We have to remember that the early almoners were children of their time, of the Victorian era: they subscribed to the values of their day. Miss Cummins (appointed lady almoner to St Thomas' Hospital in 1905) was a Victorian lady to the core and felt it to be her moral duty to encourage thrift. She wrote in one of her reports:

It is hard to contend against the increasing desire displayed on all sides to adopt the short-sighted policy of feeding both mothers and babies gratuitously in a wholesale manner. Such a policy must tend to lessen parental responsibility and undermine the value of 'backbone and grit' in family life . . . . When, as is often the case, the father of the family spends his money on betting and drink and does not work because he is lazy it is absolutely wrong to step in and support the mother or child. The responsibility for such cases rests neither with the hospital nor with the charitable agency but with the man himself.

She does confess that 'it is hard and at times almost heartbreaking to withhold the so-called help'. Miss L. C. Marx, who quotes these lines in an article written in 1953, comments that they 'read strangely today'.[3] We, living in 1990 may no longer find these words so strange. One may, perhaps, here quote Professor J. K. Galbraith:

This great centuries-old tradition is to argue that any form of public help to the poor only hurts the poor. It destroys morale. It seduces people away from gainful employment. There is no real proof of this – none certainly that compares that damage to the damage that would

be inflicted by the loss of public assistance. Still, the case is made
– and believed. There is something gravely damaging about aid to
the unfortunate. It is perhaps our most highly influential piece of
fiction.[4]

In 1903 the Hospital Almoners' Association was formed by
the working almoners, and a committee of this association
formulated the Almoners' duties as follows:

1. To reduce the number of casualty patients (an early cause
    of friction with the medical profession, this, as the medical
    and surgical staff objected that it 'tended to limit the out-
    patients and thus militated against the excellence of teaching
    material').
2. To interview patients to discover if the doctor's advice can
    be satisfactorily followed. (The emphasis is on the patient,
    not the need of the hospital.)
3. To encourage thrift.

Contrast this with the duties laid down by the hospital board
for Miss C. M. Marx, who was appointed to the Great Northern
Central Hospital (now the Royal Northern) in 1906:

1. To be at the hospital daily from 9.30 a.m. to 5 p.m.
2. To carry out a scheme for the admission of out-patients.
3. To assist the Ladies' Committee with the distribution of the
    Samaritan Fund.
4. To register all out-patients and take care of the register
    and records. (Yes, the first almoners were also the first
    administrators in the hospitals. They took on the task,
    feeling that muddle leads to patient distress, but handed
    over to trained administrators at the first opportunity.)
5. To keep a register of in-patients and make all enquiries about
    in-patients required by the House Committee.
6. To carry out such duties as may be allotted to her by the
    Committee.

The hospital authorities mainly wanted an administrator,
someone who could bring order to the chaos of the out-patients
departments of the time, and who could also stop 'abuse' of the
free treatment given by the charitable institution, the hospital.
Interestingly enough, the almoners discovered that in fact there
was very little real abuse of out-patients departments and Miss
Stewart reported:

There seems to be very little intentional imposition, probably not more than three or four, at the outside, of the 150 patients seen who could afford a private practitioner for any lengthened attendance, but on the other hand a large number could on their own showing contribute a small sum regularly to a Provident Medical Association.[5]

In spite of all the weeding-out the medical social workers did, out-patients departments remained overcrowded places well into the late 1940s and early 1950s, with anxious people milling about or meekly waiting for they knew not what, babies bawling, toddlers toddling under foot, and nurses bustling about with medical notes and X-rays. The social worker's 'office' might be a partitioned-off corner of the out-patients' hall, where confidentiality was guaranteed by the din going on around. It was still expected that the almoner interviewed most out-patients at least once, at their first attendance, and thereafter at need (as perceived by the patient or the almoner, or both). At present the hospital social worker's task seems to have shifted mainly to the wards, and out-patients is a quieter place. This is possibly because everybody now has access to a general practitioner and the help and services from health visitors and district nurses.

As early as 1906 it was realised that almoners needed a systematic training. Before this they had all worked for the COS before becoming hospital almoners. Their training included theoretical study of relevant social subjects, as well as practical case work and experience in existing almoners' departments. The COS advised the hospitals as to suitable candidates for appointments. The link between the almoners and the COS remained throughout, and trainee hospital social workers always had a three-month full-time placement with the COS (FWA).

In 1906 the Hospital Almoners' Council was formed. Its functions were defined as follows:

1. To draw up a scheme of training for hospital almoners.
2. To select candidates for training and to supervise their studies.
3. To promote the appointment of competent almoners.

In 1922 this body became the Institute of Hospital Almoners, incorporated, and continued to exist side by side with the Hospital Almoners' Association, which had been formed by the seven first almoners 'to discuss the possibilities and difficulties of the work'. In 1944, when the Association had 600 members and the Institute 120 students in training, it was decided to fuse the two and the Institute of Almoners was born in 1945. It was renamed the Institute of Medical Social Workers in 1963. The Institute's duties were to train almoners, to advise hospitals about suitable candidates for posts, to negotiate salaries, to maintain standards and to undertake research. From 1927 onwards it published a monthly journal with notes and news and articles on the different specialities within medical social work.

Until 1915 there was a slow but steady growth in the numbers of almoners appointed. They widened the scope of the work; for instance, having identified the need for health education and providing the means for healthy living, they set about supplying it. Even as early as 1907 we read in a record of the proceedings of the Hospital Almoners' Council, of 'steps to be taken to ensure a safe supply of milk for infants'. On another occasion, during a meeting of the Hospital Almoners' Association, a member 'submitted a card of advice to mothers intended to contain such information as is essential to the satisfactory rearing of children. The card was discussed and approved and it was suggested to be sold to intelligent mothers at a cost of one penny.' As social workers they knew the conditions people lived under in the community outside the hospital walls, and they did a great deal of home visiting, teaching people about the need for good food, fresh air (tuberculosis was rife and rickets was 'the scourge of the working population' as Miss Mud described in her first report to the Leeds General Infirmary Committee in 1910) and to discourage people from swaddling their babies. Miss Cummins describes in one of her reports how babies wore 'binders' – a yard long strip of cotton or flannel, tightly wound round the body; the winding could be done by laying the binder on the floor and rolling the baby round and round into it. Almoners thus were the pioneers of health visiting, a task later handed over to the specially trained health visitors.

1.1.2 1920s and 1930s

Because of the depression, the hospitals found that their bene-factors could no longer meet the growing demands from a public increasingly aware of the advantages of treatment, and patients were asked to pay. The social workers foresaw that this could cause great hardship, and might force people to put off coming for treatment until it was perhaps too late, so the Almoners' Association felt that financial assessment of patients, to determine how much they would have to pay, had better be done by the almoners, to ensure that the money was 'justly and considerately raised through knowledge of social conditions and of the prognosis of the disease'.[6] They caused a great deal of trouble for themselves, taking on this task, many of them being appointed solely for the purpose of dealing with money, and becoming associated in the public mind with financial assessment. The public saw the almoner as someone who tried to collect as much money as possible and membership in a hospital contributory scheme was advertised as offering great advantage to members because they would be immune 'from the interrogation of the Almoner'. By 1928 almoners were well aware of the dangers of their position and often discussed 'the best method of making the public realise that an almoner should not primarily be appointed to collect money, but to do social work.' As we shall see they were more successful in this than they realised at the time, even though local newspapers published, under the heading: 'The inquisition of the almoner', a list of weekly assessments. In a novel written in 1938 we come across the following passage, where one hospital patient gives another 'one sound piece of advice': '"See here, chum," he said hoarsely, "you want to watch that Miss MacMahon. She'll try an' make you pay for what they done to you, but don't you do it. If you got any o'the dibs, don't let on, see? . . ." 'Warren gathered that Miss MacMahon must be the Almoner,'[7] Later on in the novel it transpires that Miss MacMahon has some quite sound ideas about the connections between unemployment, poverty, state of mind and illness. However, even as late as 1943 a letter-writer to a newspaper hoped that 'the Almoner would go with the coming of Beveridge'. In fact, the notion persists till this day, even among the almoner's inheritors:

Hospitals are about loss, and adjustment to loss. In the old days the Lady Almoner's job was to ascertain how much patients could reasonably contribute towards their pre-NHS keep. Hospital Social Workers today see this as a strange heritage.[8]

In spite of the administrative pressures on them – they had to assess every single patient who came for treatment and had to arrange convalescence, order surgical appliances and apply for extra nourishment – the social workers kept their interest in social work alive and by the late 1920s they became more interested in 'psychological work' as practised in the United States in child-guidance clinics. Some almoners went to the States to study and almoner students were given a three-month training course at the Maudsley Hospital. They always tried to keep their clients' body and soul together by assisting them with emotional support as well as material help.

1.1.3 The Second World War

The outbreak of the Second World War brought a great deal of confusion and the Institute of Almoners thought that training would have to be suspended for the duration, so that would-be students could serve the country in different ways, and some almoners were informed by their hospital management committees that they were no longer required. Every hospital in the country swung overnight into the Emergency Medical Service and a social service was considered to be a luxury. However, things turned out differently: by Christmas 1939 the Institute was back in business and in fact training expanded and was refined during the war. An Emergency Medical Service circular advised hospitals to retain certain personnel, a list of which included almoners – almoners' posts having been classified among the reserved occupations by the Ministry of Labour – and the Minister of Health would 'recognise any reasonable amount paid in salary [to a qualified almoner] as properly incurred under the Emergency Health Scheme'. The Ministry of Health issued a circular in December 1940 which stated:

In the Minister's opinion, it is essential that a person who is a qualified almoner or has had experience in almoner's work should be employed in that capacity in all hospitals which admit a substantial number of EMS patients; in the larger hospitals it may be necessary to appoint more than one to do this work . . . . The duties which the almoner would perform are much wider than the assessment of contributions from certain classes of patients . . . and extend over the whole range of services which a trained or experienced almoner renders towards the social welfare and after-care of patients.

The need for the services of an almoner is accentuated by the problems created by air bombardment. For instance, it should be the duty of this officer (especially in the peripheral hospitals) to discover, before patients are discharged, whether their homes have been destroyed or damaged by bombing, so that alternative arrangements may be made when discharge to the patients' homes is undesirable.[9]

Discharge planning has remained an important part of the hospital social worker's task. In the early 1950s in London these social workers still interviewed, for instance, all the mothers of children being admitted for tonsillectomy, to discover their home conditions. If the home sounded totally unsuitable, a home visit would be made. Often whole families or lonely and desperately sick people were still to be found living in the basements of bomb-damaged houses in unspeakable conditions. Convalescence would then be arranged for children after treatment, even after such a relatively minor operation as tonsillectomy, so that they could gain the strength to withstand the home environment! At the present time hospital social workers arrange home-care packages for the elderly and help many other patients make plans for their discharge, still a vital task to ensure that the benefit of hospital treatment is not lost.

The Beveridge Committee started in spring 1940 to collect material and to plan for the reorganisation of health care in a post-war Britain which resulted in the creation of the National Health Service in July 1948. Training at the Institute expanded rapidly during this time, as there was a shortage of almoners, and the profession would not accept the employment of untrained workers.

1.1.4 The almoner's role under the NHS

In September 1948 a memorandum issued by the Ministry of Health stated that the almoner's duties should properly include the following:

1. Social investigation and interviews to provide understanding of the social and personal background of the patient, and in particular to give the doctor information which is relevant to diagnosis and treatment.
2. Social action to minimise personal anxieties, family difficulties and other problems during illness.
3. The making of arrangements with the Local Health Authorities

concerned for the home visiting of patients who may for a time, or in some instances for a long period, need help to ensure that the value of their treatment is not lost.[10]

The Ministry also pointed out that the almoner's department should be a focal point for teaching on social questions for student doctors and nurses. 'It is therefore specially important that their services should be confined to tasks for which they have special qualifications and that they should have such clerical or administrative assistance as may be necessary.'

Those almoners who agonised over the seeming impossibility of impressing on people the fact that they were not primarily concerned with the raising of money, must have been overjoyed to see themselves at long last accepted as social workers. The coming of the National Health Service freed them from much of the administrative and money raising work that had occupied most of their time in previous decades and was hailed with relief and delight. Dorothy Manchée tells aspiring almoners of the importance of raising money from charitable sources to supply a woman suffering from stomach ulcers with a set of false teeth.[11] They had to raise money for corsets, wigs and convalescence. All these things were henceforth to be available on the NHS, and social workers could at last concentrate on social work (helping people with the giving of much needed facts, simple, accurate information, welfare rights advice and practical help) and what was then called case-work, and nowadays counselling (notably crisis counselling, bereavement counselling and family therapy), the element in social work which many social workers based in hospital would still see as their most arduous and most important task as well as the one which gives them most job satisfaction. However, it was not to last and social workers find themselves once again writing to charities to raise money for convalescence and help parents find the money for fares to visit their sick children in hospital. With the implementation of the recent White Paper, *Caring for People*, we may well come full circle, as the 'assessment of individuals' needs' will include financial assessment. Many social workers now advance the same arguments for taking on this task as the almoners did: to ensure that money is 'justly and considerately raised through knowledge of social conditions and of the prognosis of the disease'.

From 1948 onwards most almoners' departments – the Institute changed its name to the Institute of Medical Social Workers
in 1963 and the hospitals henceforth had medical social work
departments – were run on the lines suggested by the Ministry
of Health and most teaching hospitals and many non-teaching
hospitals up and down the country had such a department.
The head social worker was in full charge and did her own
hiring and firing.[12] They managed the hospital's Samaritan
Fund, which filled gaps left by welfare state provision and
ran their own administration. They jealously guarded their
independence from the medical profession; the Cope Committee
on Medical Auxiliaries (1951), while stating that 'the work of the
almoner should be regarded as one of the essential elements of
a complete hospital service, and indeed of a complete health
service', assumed that they must be medical auxiliaries, which
meant that doctors could and should plan and control the
training of and methods used by medical social workers. The
Institute of Almoners refused to accept this and the social
workers never became medical auxiliaries and remained an
independent profession.

The Institute tried to clarify what were the duties of medical
social workers, particularly during the 1950s and 1960s. They
commissioned a number of surveys and research projects,[13] and
worked hard to help medical social workers to shed administrative duties that still clung to them for historical reasons,
like supplying appliances and arranging transport for patients.
An Institute report stated that:

The almoner is essentially the medical social worker whose job it is to
study the patient's social background and his reactions to illness, with
a view to assisting in the solution of the many personal and practical
problems which are associated with illness .... Problems which
require listening, helping the patient to sort out worrying situations,
to face the future and possible readjustments to his life or the
limitations of his disability can only be dealt with by the medical
social worker .... The almoner will also be required to arrange for
a wide variety of practical forms of help for patients.[14]

Training by the Institute took nine months, which included a
three-month full-time placement at the Family Welfare Association, and was undertaken only by people with relevant degrees,
or the equivalent, thereby having become in effect a post-

graduate course. It must be admitted that, as many social workers in other fields did not have a unified training and registration, or a body to set standards and defend their position, medical social workers rather felt themselves to be an elite amongst social workers, admitting only that perhaps the psychiatric social workers were of a similar standing!

During the 1960s the Institute became active in promoting a unified social work professional association, through regional and university social work staffs, and when they changed their name in 1963 they commented that 'the out-of-date title of almoner created an artificial barrier between medical social workers and the wider field of social work to which they belong by virtue of their training as well as by the nature, aims and methods of their work'.[15]

The Younghusband Report (which reported on the need for a unified training scheme for social workers in 1959) foreshadowed the Seebohm Report (1968) in that it called for a 'general purpose social worker' with a two-year training. They reported on social workers in the health and welfare services and in particular did not like the division along the lines of physical and mental handicap. Obviously, from this time onwards much has been written and there have been many discussions about the future of the social services and the training and employment of social workers, beyond the scope of the present work. Suffice it to say that after Seebohm the 'generic' social worker was born and in 1974 the local authorities took over the responsibility for providing a social work service to hospitals from the NHS. The NHS however, was and still is responsible for supplying the social work departments in hospitals with clerical services, office supplies and accommodation. The Institute of Medical Social Workers ceased to exist in 1974 and merged with the British Association of Social Workers. Specialist training was no longer available and generically trained social workers gained their special knowledge on the job, in the hospitals.

1.2 Recurring issues

1.2.1 Wider horizons

Medical social workers had for many years called for the placement of social workers in general medical practices, and at the time of the reorganisation in 1974 hopes were high that experienced hospital social workers would be employed in community health centres; the majority of people, after all, suffer their illnesses outside the hospital, and may well be in as great a need of social work help as those admitted to the hospital. Generic area teams are not often equipped with sufficient social workers aware of the special needs of sick and disabled people and their carers to deal with the problems that arise through sickness, old age, disability and death in the community. In any case, their time and attention is fully taken up by the needs of children and families.

In some social services departments 'disability teams' are being created, but this still does not provide support for sick people, or dying people, or those who come to their general practitioners with physical complaints which have a psychological origin, or who are addicted to tranquillisers. The report *Social Work Support for the Health Service* stated:

We hope that all new health centres will be designed to include accommodation for the use of social workers . . . . Generally, we see development of support for general practice as a priority for the future, since it presents a major opportunity for significant improvement in methods of health and social care.[16]

Social workers based in health centres could do a great deal of preventive work and help turn them into true *health* centres, rather than *sickness* centres, as they may be at present. There are however, few permanent, full-time attachments of social workers to general practices. Research has been done, experimental attachments have been made, but so far most GPs have not asked for social work support, many of them being unaware of the help social workers could give them and their patients. Another problem being the permanent shortage of well-trained workers experienced in hospital social work, and the money to employ them.

It is to be hoped that 'disaster teams', now being set up in many parts of the country, will make full use of the expertise of hospital-based social workers, whose daily work consists mainly of crisis intervention and bereavement counselling of people who have never seen a social worker before, and never expected themselves to need the help of one.

Generic social workers may have little experience of 'selling' social work to those people who see social workers as dealing only with the 'mad, bad and inadequate', who would feel that being visited by 'the welfare' carries with it a social stigma. Sickness, and 'disaster, like death itself, cares little about our social agendas',[17] they are no respectors of persons, class or social status. Michael Stewart discusses the problems social workers encountered when trying to counsel people coming to terms with the aftermath of disasters like the Bradford fire (see also Chapter 3). It might help if such teams could operate from local hospitals: people find it easier to accept help which is offered as from a hospital than that offered as from a social work department.

1.2.2 The expectations of the institution

As we have seen the first medical social workers were appointed, or accepted by the hospital in the expectation that they would bring order out of administrative chaos, and at the same time save them money. In order to gain a foothold in an institution, which badly needed a social work presence, the almoners did what was expected of them and at the same time attempted to do work which they saw as even more important: social work and health education. But they were not able to be vocal enough about what they saw as their true sphere of work, and often felt frustrated and undervalued. In a way they created this pitfall for themselves by being good administrators and doing financial assessments. It was done with the best of motives: to minimise distress to patients, but as far as the institution was concerned, they earned their keep by minimising inconvenience to it.

Almoners cleared the out-patients departments, as there were too many patients for too few facilities. Nowadays the problem lies with in-patients: too many for too few beds, and social workers are expected to help clear beds as speedily as possible. (If they value their relationship with the medical profession, they had better not be too efficient in this: we read in the Oxfordshire Health Authority District Short Term Programme 1988/89, p. 65: 'Too many doctors and students are at the present chasing insufficient experience. Too few patients are in long enough to provide for careful study.' Sounds familiar!) The pressure on social workers to get on with clearing beds is not entirely a phenomenon of the 1980s: an article in *Medical Social Work*, the Institute Journal, dated January 1967, is entitled: 'Social worker or disposal unit?'.

Once again they are expected to find out if the patients can afford the treatment needed, this time it is usually a matter of paying for private long-term care (some NHS hospitals no longer provide long-stay beds), so that they do not block beds in free hospitals. Social workers are then expected to help patients and their relatives make financial arrangements with private nursing homes, which now proliferate all over the country. The hospitals are being pressurised to be 'efficient', to have a quick turnover of patients and social workers are asked to arrange for patients to vacate the beds as soon as immediate medical needs are dealt with. We should be clear at all times about what we think social work proper is, and to aim at fulfilling that role rather than one thrust upon us by hospital authorities. Certainly, muddle in out-patients, as in the past, and too early discharges, which may happen nowadays, cause distress and suffering to patients, and may negate the work done by the other professionals in the hospital and social workers may therefore feel compelled to help sort things out. Almoners learned to do tasks which were not, in their eyes their primary duty, but which were to the benefit of patients. They were also extremely good at handing these tasks over to others when the time was ripe. They handed administration over to administrators, and health education and visiting to health visitors. It behoves us to learn from their clear-eyed pursuit of their objective: a social work department devoted to social work.

1.2.3 Communication with medical staff

As we have seen, at the beginning of the hospital social work service social workers incurred the wrath of the medical profession by being too efficient in weeding out patients who should not be (according to the standards of the time) attending the hospital's out-patients department at all. The medical profession had not asked for this and to an extent social workers have remained a 'foreign body' in the hospital. In the States the need for medical social workers to deal with the psycho-social needs of patients was seen by the medical profession itself (notably Dr

Richard Cabot), which made it easier for them to fulfil the role of the true social worker and for them to be accepted and used to their full potential; although at present their work seems in some respects to have much in common with pre-NHS social work practice in that they have to maintain clothing cupboards, see that out-patients get food, etc.[18] In Britain, however, despite the lack of support from the medical profession (almoner students often discussed the difficulties of 'educating the doctors'!) hospital social workers saw themselves as linking body and mind.

However, the main problem is one of communication. Communication is hindered by the following:

1. In this country the medical profession has, on the whole, tended to concentrate on the mechanics of the human body. They have, perhaps, been encouraged in this by the prevailing climate of opinion, that the sciences are more valuable and have a higher standing in society than the humanities – even literary critics are trying to be more scientific in their approach, in order to gain prestige – and the medical profession would, it seems likely, be offended if someone suggested that the practice of medicine is more of an art than a science. The whole of society tends to value the scientific doctor above the social worker, whose whole existence is based on the humanities. It is therefore still as difficult for the social worker to do her work and gain respect and credence in the hospital setting as it is elsewhere in the community. When writing reports for medical notes, and communicating verbally with medics, social workers have to use spare, unemotional language, as close to a scientific language as possible in order to be heard and taken seriously. Social workers are being asked to prove they are cost-effective, to provide statistics of 'positive or negative outcomes' of their intervention. This is scientific jargon and tries to apply scientific criteria to a non-scientific endeavour.

2. In the traditional, hierarchical structure of the hospital the doctor, or consultant, has always been seen as being in charge and directing the activities of the other professionals working there. Social workers have kept their independence, are not medical auxiliaries, and are even employed by a different

authority. They are therefore not under the consultants' direction. This can cause difficulties for consultants, who have to work with someone whose activities they cannot control or direct as has been traditional in the hospital setting. Neither can the social worker direct them. It can happen that the consultant says: 'this patient will be discharged tomorrow, there is nothing further I can offer her'. The social worker may have to say: 'no, the patient can not be discharged, the community support is not yet in place'. It then depends on their working relationship and ease of communication who wins, or what kind of compromise is achieved.

3. There is a basic difference in approach to the patient or client between the medical profession and social workers. Doctors traditionally see themselves, and are seen by the patient as the experts who can tell what is wrong and what must be done to put it right, to *prescribe*, sometimes without much time for thought, when the matter is an urgent one of life or death. Social workers however, are taught never to know what is good for their client, but to help her come to her own decision and determine her own fate. Their methods strike members of the health professions as slow and indecisive. This difference in attitude to patients can make communication and understanding between the professions difficult indeed. As Bywaters says:

> Social work finds itself at odds with medicine in its central belief in a respect for the client's self-knowledge and right to choice, and in its growing recognition of the value of mutual support and exchange. Medical expectations of patient passivity fit uneasily with social work objectives of a self-directed and empowered clientele.[19]

The social worker needs to be able to gain trust and respect from the people belonging to other professions in the hospital and to be prepared to spend time on building relationships within the institution, so as to overcome any communication difficulties which may exist. Her predecessors, the almoners, did it, albeit slowly and painfully and they found their contribution to patient care fully acknowledged at various stages, notably during the Second World War, and at the beginning of the Health Service. Let us hope that present and future generations of hospital-based social workers will learn from their example and ensure that sick people get the services they need in order to recover, that dying people and their families are given counselling where necessary, and that handicapped people are enabled to take as full a part as they are capable of in the life of our community, and their carers are sustained in their task.

Notes

1. As quoted in: Manchée, Dorothy, *Textbook for Almoners*, London: Bailliere, Tindall & Cox, 1947, p. 3.
2. *ibid.*, p. 4.
3. Marx, L. C., 'Early days', *The Almoner*, Golden Jubilee number, November 1953.
4. Galbraith, J. K., 'Poverty and society', *Community Care*, 23 February 1989.
5. Beck, I. F., *The Almoner*, Institute of Almoners, undated.
6. Edmonson, M. W., 'The Middle Period, or Episode Two', *The Almoner*, November 1953.
7. Shute, Nevil, *Ruined City*, London: Heinemann, 1938.
8. Dickinson, Jennifer, 'Through the knife-edge hours', *The Guardian*, 5 April 1989, p. 27.
9. Ministry of Health Circular 2232, December 1940.
10. HMC (48)53; BG 48(57).
11. Manchée, Dorothy, *Social Service in a General Hospital*, London: Bailliere, Tindall & Cox, 1943.
12. Most medical social workers were women.
13. e.g. Marjorie Moon and Kathleen Slack, *The First Two Years*, Institute of Medical Social Workers, 1965.
14. Institute of Almoners, Survey Report, 1953.
15. Quoted in: Younghusband, Eileen, *Social Work in Britain: 1950–1975*, London: George Allen & Unwin, 1978, p. 148.
16. *Social Work Support for the Health Service*, London: HMSO, 1974, p. 66.
17. Stewart, Michael, 'Crisis counselling – Selling social work', *Community Care*, 9 February 1989.
18. Suskis, Carole W., *Social Work in the Emergency Room*, New York: Spurger, 1985.
19. Bywaters, Paul, 'Social work and the medical profession – Arguments against unconditional collaboration'. *British Journal of Social Work*, **16**, 1986, p. 670.

Suggestions for further reading

Beck, Flora, *Ten Patients and an Almoner*, London: George Allen & Unwin, 1956.

Clare, Anthony, and Corney, Roslyn (eds), *Social Work and Primary Health Care*, London: Academic Press, 1982.

Huntington, June, *Social Work and General Medical Practice, Collaboration or Conflict?*, London: George Allen & Unwin, 1981.

CHAPTER 2

The organisation of social work in a Health Service setting

JEAN CARR AND NIGEL PARSONS

This chapter considers the significant influences in the management of a social work service in a hospital setting: what hospital social workers do and arising from that, why social workers should be placed in hospital settings; how social workers could be managed, and how this structure can initiate and extend the joint working between health and social services departments on a wider level. It is important to consider hospital social work as part of the total working relationship between these two statutory authorities in which significant changes are taking place at present. Factors currently influencing the services provided by both authorities are significant developments in medical practice; the location of social services fieldwork provisions; the White Papers *Working for Patients* and *Caring for People*, on the provision and funding of health and community care; and the development of relationships between health and social services and the voluntary sector.

The future of social work in hospitals cannot be considered separately from the future of social work in social services departments and the changing expectations of the roles and tasks of social workers. This is a time of considerable changes and developments in the functions of local authorities and the National Health Service; it is therefore an opportunity to step outside established attitudes and ask again how services should be provided and managed to give the best possible service to people facing trauma caused by illness. The post-war social services were organised to meet specific problems in client groups, hence the development of children's departments, mental health departments and welfare departments. They were geared to look at specific problems, rather than to look at the needs of a family as a whole and the social circumstances in which they were living in an effort to prevent family breakdown. Consideration should now be given to learning from the past and discarding models that may not meet the best interests of the client.

2.1 Organisational changes

The Seebohm Committee recommended a local authority department 'providing a community-based and family-orientated service, which will be available to all'.[1] This was to be achieved through amalgamating separate departments into a larger unified organisation, reducing fragmentation and duplication of existing services and thus creating a powerful focus for resources. These departments, set up in the early 1970s and expanded between 1971 and 1974, developed the supervisory and managerial structures required for larger and more complex organisations. However, there was little or no management training of existing staff for these new responsibilities.

Since then social workers have also been out-posted in other settings, for example in general practice, with the police, attached to various drug and alcohol treatment services and a variety of other settings to ensure that social work services are more directly available to clients. This theme of taking the service to the people rather than the other way round is a significant development. Thus social work in hospital has developed alongside social work in non-hospital settings, and the management of the service has been subject to similar issues and influences.

The social work task in a hospital setting covers a wide variety of situations. In some medical specialisms only a small proportion of patients will need social work help, in others, for example, in what used to be called geriatric medicine, the majority may well do so. The social worker, like social workers in area teams, may work short term in a problem-solving way, or may be involved in long-term work with family problems, or problems of adjustment to loss or a life-long illness. The level of overlap between the tasks performed by the social workers and those performed by other members of the multidisciplinary team will vary considerably, depending on the type of specialism.

The report *Social Work Support to the Health Service* (1974) outlines that the social worker has a contribution to make to the work of the clinical team at various stages:

1. *Diagnosis*: An assessment of the social factors involved may be an essential contribution to diagnosis and this is a task in which social workers are much involved.
2. *Treatment*: Decisions on the best method of treatment where alternatives are available sometimes depend as much on social as on medical considerations. Medical services . . . may be ineffective or reduced in benefit to the patient if [they are] delivered without consideration of his way of life and his potential for adaptation in social terms.
3. *Discharge*: Decisions about timing and arrangements for discharge should be made in full knowledge of the social as well as the medical situation of the patient. This can be a stressful time, especially after a long period in hospital, or if the patient has to face changes as a result of illness or handicap. In some cases help may be required long after discharge from a hospital ward. Attempted suicide, abortions, non-accidental injury to children, alcohol and drug abuse are all examples of situations where medical attention may be short term, but where the crisis has revealed a need for extensive social rehabilitation and therapy. Social workers share the task of providing long-term support for such patients with general practitioners, health visitors and community nurses.[2]

2.2 Advantages of having social workers in health settings

One of the most significant advantages of social workers in a hospital setting is their contribution to the multidisciplinary team. A well-functioning multidisciplinary team is much more than the sum of its parts, and development of teamwork can be a difficult although rewarding process. Matilda Goldberg and June Neal write in *Social Work in General Practice* that individual members of the team widen their concept of their professional skills and discover new delineations of roles.[3] They also became more comfortable about interchange of functions, and adopt more flexible and imaginative attitudes towards the areas of client need, which are characteristically vague in primary medical care. At the same time everyone becomes sharply aware of their individual skills.

The needs of people referred to hospital and area teams are similar. However, the role of individual social workers is determined by the type of team of which they are a member and the population they serve. Area based social workers serve a geographical population made up of people with varying degrees of medical and social problems. The population served by hospital social workers are all those who attend the hospital for in-patient, out-patient and emergency treatment throughout a given year. This population is therefore determined by individual health needs and not their home address. In a recent study it was noted that about one-third of the clients with whom social workers were working were found to have social problems arising solely from health-related factors, that is to say, had they not become ill there would have been no reason for social work involvement. In the remaining two-thirds of referrals, pre-existing factors were seen either as the main area of the client's problems, exacerbated by health-related factors, thus creating a more complex background for social work intervention.[4]

It is important to consider not only what hospital social workers do, but why they should be based and managed in hospitals. There is a need for social workers to be available in places where people with problems go for help, and it is to general practitioners and hospitals that people go for help with not only their medical problems but also general social and personal problems. In 1986 NHS provision treated 6.4 million in-patient cases, 37.4 million out-patient attendances, and 12.8 million accident and emergency attendances. The majority of these people were experiencing a crisis in their lives. Illness and social functioning are intimately bound up with each other, and require expert assessment to provide appropriate help addressing both factors. It is only when both are correctly diagnosed and effectively treated that the person can make progress. Social workers in hospitals therefore need to acquire the general knowledge base for social work practice plus more detailed knowledge of illness, symptoms, likely outcome of various conditions and the effect of those physical conditions on emotional well-being.

Hospital social workers can be based and managed in the hospital setting in community teams maintaining regular contact with the hospital, or based in the hospital but managed by the community team. There is probably no one correct organisation or model, different systems being more appropriate in different parts of the country. Factors to be taken into account are the urban/rural nature of the area, the pattern and type of hospital provision and the existing arrangement for multidisciplinary work.

The need for staff in health and social services to work more closely together, as envisaged in White Paper *Caring for People*, would indicate the need to strengthen present arrangements for collaborative working at all levels. Case management as outlined in the White Paper is an extension of the present role of social workers in hospitals and, taken alongside the proposed transfer of all funding for residential placements to the local authority, will increase the importance of hospital social work.

2.3 Hospital social work tasks

The Barclay report suggested that social workers need to carry out two different but interdependent activities.[5] The first is to plan, establish, maintain and evaluate the provision of social care, the report call this 'social care planning', and saw it as an activity that needs to be practised by both social workers and their managers. The second task which social workers need to undertake is that of direct communication with their clients to help them adjust to changes in their lives caused through ill health. It is also useful to compare the management of hospital-based social work with managerial functions outlined in the Barclay Report. This suggested there should be the greatest possible delegation of decision-making to front-line workers as occurs when social workers are members of multidisciplinary teams. They also recommend that team leaders should retain both administrative and social work responsibilities. There has been an increasing move in the last few years towards the concept of senior practitioners and away from a structure in which client contact takes place only through front-line workers. Hospital social workers often maintain client contact when they move into more supervisory positions. In the National Health Service, senior people in most disciplines maintain a high level of practice, as well as supervisory and management responsibilities. In this way they can keep up to date with developments in practice, and ensure that patients are seen by staff with experience, and not only by new recruits.

The Seebohm Report recommended that social workers should be attached on a fairly long-term basis to institutions such as schools, health centres, courts and hospitals, while continuing to be employed by social services departments. If this were to be implemented on any substantial basis, it could undermine the area team as the current focal point of social work intervention. Basing social work services in other settings does present some problems both to the managers and to individual workers who are working alongside other disciplines with a wide variety of professional attitudes and practices. Also, social workers in isolated positions in other settings can lack the support provided by close association with colleagues. Managers can be more distant from detailed knowledge of the workers' referrals and performance, and have to establish a different working relationship with the managers and professionals in other settings, for example head teachers, consultants, etc. Social workers do not have a monopoly on caring and helping people, other professionals also do this, often in a different way, but certainly with no less effectiveness and with no less motivation. Some managers in social services departments are uneasy about having social workers located outside traditional area teams who are arguably less responsive to their control and potentially subject to the influences of other disciplines. However, a skilled social worker can establish independence of practice, while promoting the values of social work, which can then positively influence and redress any imbalance that might exist in the power relationship between the health authority and the patient, for example in planning for hospital discharge.

2.4 Organisational links

As well as the value of social workers attached to multi-disciplinary teams in the provision of a range of services to the patient, this structure provides an important link between the health authority and social services department. Hospital social workers can identify the changes in Health Service practice which have implications for social services departments and can assist both organisations in finding the appropriate channels for communication. Hospital social workers therefore function at this significant boundary between the two statutory organisations who are most responsible for providing services for people in need. Work at any boundary can be difficult and anxiety producing and the management of the service must take these factors into account. The pattern of service provision in the future is increasingly towards a multitude of organisations and agencies being responsible for providing services, with the consequent problems associated with agencies with different priorities and values working together. Hospital social workers and their managers have a contribution to make to the discussion on how different agencies can work together to provide an integrated and comprehensive service for people in need. The Griffiths Report, commissioned by central government to consider the cost of community care,[6] has led to a wide debate at central and local government level on how community care can be provided in the most cost effective and consumer orientated way.

2.5 Departmental priorities within the hospital setting

With the benefits of social workers placed in hospital settings come various problems as identified in the Audit Commission Report 1986 which identifies the difficulties of setting priorities in a health service.[7] Where staff are directly responsible for accepting referrals, as in a hospital setting, it can be difficult to establish priorities for work taken on. They must, for example, balance caseloads, maintain consistent practice and implement the department's overall strategy for work with particular client groups. Social workers in hospital tend to work in specialist areas making it more difficult to respond to changes in priorities between the different client groups. However, a specialist service is essential if one is to develop and keep up to date with a complex knowledge base. Managers must therefore achieve a balance between work in specialist areas and the key priorities of the social services department. Those priorities identified in the DHSS circular on Rate Fund Expenditure issued in 1974 are just as valid today.[8] They are as follows:

1. Children at risk of ill treatment.
2. The very elderly or severely handicapped person living alone,

especially those discharged from hospital, recently bereaved or in inadequate housing.
3. The mentally handicapped or mentally ill in urgent need of residential day care or domiciliary support, to prevent deterioration of their condition and to relieve intolerable strain on their families.
4. Individuals or families with vulnerable members who are at imminent risk of breakdown under severe stress, imposed upon them by handicap, illness, homelessness or poverty.

It is important that the priority areas of work undertaken by hospital social workers are those of the social services department, but when working in multidisciplinary teams, where members of several different professions come together, social workers are subject to the pressures and priorities of other members of the team, and vice versa.

2.6 Structures for hospital social work

Various structures have been developed for hospital social work. From studies and experiences across the country, it would seem that no system can be considered ideal and suited to all circumstances. One key issue is whether social services departments and the health authority are responsible for the same geographic area. In London, where there are many large teaching hospitals serving the whole of London with national catchment areas, there are considerable difficulties in the resources of one local authority being used to provide a service for residents from others. As yet no way of cross-charging for these services has been found, and this has led to a considerable drain on the resources of those authorities so affected and has led to hospital social work services on occasions being disbanded. Health services have developed in different ways around the country. One county can have the majority of its health services focused in a centre of a population, whereas another may have hospitals spread across it. Local geography, the location of hospitals and the structure of the social services department are some of the factors to be taken into account in deciding the best social services managerial structure for a given area. No one structure can be the optimum for all circumstances. There are implications for both workers and their managers resulting from out-posting. The manager must be able to support the workers, link their work into the social services department, and be familiar with the setting in which that work is carried out. Management needs to relate not only to the health services that are provided in the hospital, but also to community services provided outside. Much of a hospital-based social worker's work can be with patients who have been discharged, or who have never been in-patients.

2.7 *Managing hospital social work*

Apart from operational accountability, managers of hospital social workers are in a unique position to identify issues in both health and social services departments and to enable better communication to take place between the two organisations. This function of management has become increasingly significant with the pressures on the Health Service and the closure of hospital beds, creating additional pressures on local authority services. One measure of efficiency in the Health Service is throughput and mortality, as these are objective measures that can be easily collected, validated and compared across the country. A more efficient health service measured by greater throughput, however, can lead to significant problems for individual patients and their relatives, and can also create considerable pressures on social services departments.

Developing a comprehensive package of community care is a significant part of the task of hospital social workers, and much community care planning is initiated from the hospital setting, whether it is arranging a care package for a family which has a child with severe physical and mental disabilities, or an elderly person living alone admitted to hospital after a major stroke. Perhaps the key determinant in the successful provision of community care the availability of a wide range of services, from domestic help to direct personal care, including any that could be performed by a caring relative. The majority of community care is provided by relatives supported by friends. The White Paper *Caring for People*[9] does not encourage replacement, but seeks to support this basic model. Social services departments are seen as responsible for ensuring the provision of support to primary carers, and providing a similar level of care to those without such

help. Other services currently provided by the local authority
are occupational therapy, social work and practical help such
as laundry and bathing services – the Health Service providing
community nursing services.

There may be a gap between the point in time at which a
person is medically fit for discharge and when the community
care package can be started to support them in the community.
Bridging this gap is an essential part of hospital social work
practice, and failure may result in clients remaining in hospital
unnecessarily, or being discharged to inadequate services with
insufficient support for the client and their carers.

Communication between the two authorities at all levels must
be established and maintained. The Health Service Working
Party (1974) recommended that each local authority identify
a senior officer, responsible to the director, for arranging social
work support to area health authorities, and be the point of
contact for the area health authority management within the
department. It is important that any such post has not only
operational responsibility for social workers based in hospitals,
but has a much wider brief to look at health issues generally. The
significance of health-related issues for social services practice
and organisation needs to be identified, and links between social
services departments and the health authorities developed and
maintained.

2.8 Recent developments

Currently there are a number of developments that are affecting
practice, both in social services departments and in the National
Health Service. The Audit Commission Report (1986), followed by
the Griffiths Report, outlined the issues facing the organisation of
community care services. It would seem essential that, following
the Griffiths Report, developments are made to integrate community care services provided by social services and the National
Health Service. The government's recent White Paper on the
reorganisation of the National Health Service primarily addresses
provision of acute services, saying very little about services
provided by anyone other than doctors. This report does not
address the needs of physically and mentally disabled people in
the longer term. Alongside this, there have been considerable

advances in medicine leading to many lives being saved, but with people being left with much higher levels of disability than would previously have been the case. How such people can be adequately cared for, has yet to be fully addressed.

Many more children are saved through medical technology (see Chapter 8), for example in special care baby units, and some of them are left with considerable levels of disability. Parents usually do not want to place their children in institutions, but want to look after them themselves. However, there is often an inadequate level of community support for these parents. Extended periods of home care, community nursing services overnight, or for several hours a day, which would make it possible for them to keep the handicapped child at home, are not always available. When one child in the family has a high level of dependency the needs of the other children can be overlooked or are not seen as a priority and thus are not always provided for. Satisfactory levels of community care can thus become complicated and expensive, a fact which may well be overlooked. Community care cannot be seen as the cheap option, or treated as a cost-cutting exercise.

Changes in demography have led to an increasingly elderly population and in particular, very elderly population. This 'geriatric time bomb' has been much discussed, but the implications for the allocation of both health and social services resources has not yet been fully debated. Social services departments have as their main priority services for children, especially child protection, and children in care. Health districts, on the whole, have prioritised acute services, at the expense of continuing care. There has been, and continues to be, the tendency for community care services for adults to be marginalised in both services, while it is these services that present us with the most significant challenge for providing good and comprehensive services in the community. Alongside these specific changes there has been a shift in the general attitude towards a more consumer orientated approach in the provision of services, both in health and social services. Many large hospitals have closed their long-stay beds and the current funding restrictions on the NHS are now leading to the closure of more rehabilitation beds. This has been an important development and has led to less institutionalised services, but has not been matched by the transfer of resources to the community services.

2.9 Future developments

Social work services in health care settings have developed from individually appointed almoners, through to teams of highly specialised social workers employed by local government. At present the challenge is to bring the range of social services provision into health settings, and to manage the increasingly complex boundary between the two statutory organisations most concerned with the provision of care. The management of the service is no longer only the management of social workers, each within their multidisciplinary teams, and taking an individualistic casework stance towards their work. At present and increasingly in the future with the implementation of the Griffiths Report and community care developments, hospital social work managers will be responsible for developments at the critical boundary between health and social services, and for managing one of the channels through which the services of both can be harnessed for the benefit of the individual.

Notes

1. *Report of the Committee on Local Authority and Allied Social Services* (The Seebohm Report) Cmnd 3703, London: HMSO 1968, p. 18.
2. *Social Work Support for the Health Service*, London: HMSO, 1974.
3. Goldberg, Matilda, and Neal, June, *Social Work in General Practice*, London: Allen & Unwin, 1972.
4. *Social Workers in Health Care in Hospitals*, Report by Central Research Unit for Social Work Services Group, Scottish Office, 1988.
5. *Social Workers: Their role and tasks* (The Barclay Report), Bedford Square Press, HMSO 1977.
6. *Making a Reality of Community Care*, (The Griffiths Report), London: HMSO, 1988.
7. *A Pilot Study of Social Work*, (Audit Commission Report), London: HMSO, 1986.
8. DHSS Circular LAC (74) (36) *Rate Fund Expenditure and Rate Calls in 75/76*, London: HMSO, 1974.
9. HMSO, 1989.

Suggestions for further reading

Bamford, Terry, *Managing Social Work*, London: Tavistock, 1982.

Brunel Institute of Organisation and Social Studies, *Professionals in Health and Social Services Organisations*, Uxbridge: Brunel Institute of Organisation and Social Studies, October 1976.

Harrison, Steven, *Managing the National Health Service*, London: Chapman & Hall, 1988.

Sher, Manny, and Crewe, Janet, 'The changing role of social work managers in Health Service settings', *Social Work Today*, 13: number 48, 24 August 1982.

Social Services Study Group, *Social Work and the Systematic Provision of Local Authorities Social Services*, June 1979.

CHAPTER 3

The nature of medical social work

SYLVIA STEVENSON and JUDITH UNWIN

This chapter begins by exploring why some people, trying to cope with a major illness or trauma may need specialised social work help/intervention and examining the role of the hospital social worker. It then goes into the question of working relationships with other professionals with whom the social worker is in daily contact. It attempts to give some insight into her main responsibilities and tasks, and how she goes about them – the qualities necessary to be effective in an environment as complex as a hospital; the social worker's influence on colleagues and associates; and how all of this, when she is hospital based, can alter the quality of service to patients in a positive way.

3.1 The social workers' role in hospitals

The recent spate of national and international disasters (Bradford, Zeebrugge, King's Cross, Lockerbie, etc.) has focused attention on the psychological needs of the survivors and of the families who have been bereaved. In professional circles much has been published on the nature of the work undertaken by social workers and other counsellors, and the need for a proactive approach. The needs of the helpers have been highlighted; their need for some specialist training, their need for support, their need for debriefing, etc. Medical social workers have long been aware of many of the issues these disasters have made public, e.g. the impact of trauma on individuals and families, and observe many parallels to work in an acute hospital setting. Trauma and crisis are common occurrences in hospitals. Just as life changes in a split second for those involved in a major disaster, where victims are a totally random group, so are victims of road traffic accidents. They happen at any time and in any place. Illness knows no bounds either and can strike without warning. People in hospital facing personal crises, coming to terms with loss of one kind or the other, are from the whole spectrum of society – of all ages and both sexes.

Hospital casualty departments are pick up points for domestic violence – the battered wife seeking refuge, the physically abused child needing a place of safety. The hospital is a source of possible help for people overwhelmed by stress who come in with overdoses. Deep inner conflict or anxiety can manifest itself in physical symptoms necessitating clinical investigations. Anxiety, alarm and sadness are common emotions experienced by patients and relatives. The anxiety level in an out-patient department, where new patients wait to be seen by a specialist, is almost palpable. Will their worst fears be dispelled or confirmed, will hopes be shattered? The following examples come readily to mind. On an accident service ward, parents sit hopefully by the bedside of their unconscious, head-injured daughter, who had been in a road traffic accident. They are from miles away – strangers to the city without their normal supports. They sit, stroking, talking, encouraging, willing her to respond. The parents' hopes and dreams for the future, embodied in this daughter, are about to be destroyed. In the intensive therapy unit a young graduate student finally regains consciousness to discover that he has lost a quarter of his body – his last memory is of cycling back to college after dinner with a friend. He was knocked down by a drunken driver. He wishes he were dead. His parents are shattered and stunned, but grateful that he is alive. Outside the intensive therapy unit are a family from abroad, praying together, parents who had flown in, sister, cousins, aunt. A law graduate, studying in London, returning from a day trip to Stratford with two friends has been involved in a car crash. The friends did not survive. On a medical ward lies a lady only in her mid-50s following a dense stroke which left her paralysed and unable to communicate. She is very ill and may not survive. She does survive, but needs total nursing care. Her family feel desolate and helpless.

Serious illness and major trauma which threaten loss or change cause alarm, uncertainty and stress, leading to tension and a feeling of being in crisis. People in this situation may need help and deserve it. Sometimes the help of family and friends together with the patient's own coping strategy may be sufficient, but at other times the professional support of a hospital social worker is needed if the patient is to make a satisfactory adjustment and to benefit from available resources when practical, financial and other needs become evident. In an acute general hospital setting, where crisis work is commonplace, social workers should be mindful of crisis theory which not only teaches them that if help is offered at the right time there is an opportunity for change and growth, but also emphasises the effectiveness of short-term intensive support in the initial stages of a crisis.[1]

Progressive and life-threatening illnesses have far-reaching effects on relationships and family dynamics, on financial situations, on status – indeed the ramifications and implications of ill health are far and wide and can change roles, abilities, incomes, even personalities. An early assessment of the needs of patient and family allows the patient to receive and benefit from treatment, as anxiety can and does inhibit progress, co-operation and treatment plans. From time to time patients are labelled 'difficult' and 'unco-operative'. On investigation the patient is revealed to be weighed down with anxiety or with memories of an unresolved grief or trauma which the new loss has re-awakened, and is therefore unable to be 'a good patient'.

Case example: Mr T. was a professional person in his mid-50s, who was referred about ten days after the amputation of a lower limb. He was described as being 'depressed, tearful, difficult and unco-operative'. He had a delightful family and was normally a person who coped with his own life and situation. In helping this patient, the social worker discovered that he had experienced a whole series of losses from the age of five, the last being the death of a sibling whom he had not properly mourned. The loss of his leg re-awakened memories of previous losses, particularly the death of his sibling. Mr T. responded to social work intervention and subsequently co-operated and made good use of rehabilitation. He had been taught to believe that emotion was a sign of weakness and gained much relief from being given permission to react to his loss, which was very real, and to understand the reasons for the depth of his feelings and reactions. A proactive approach was subsequently established on units in the hospital where surgery occasioned loss.

Ill health in a household, particularly if it is the 'strong' member who becomes ill, can be a breaking point for people who have never coped well.

Case example: Sheila, a 42-year-old teacher with an open, immediately likeable sunny personality, was the strong partner in her second marriage, who was devastated when she was told that she had leukaemia. She had already experienced rejection and loss – married young, her first husband left her when their daughter was two. With courage and determination plus the help and support of her parents, she re-established herself. She was rehoused by the council and returned to work to become self-supporting. She married Don, an outwardly whole, good-looking man, who gradually demonstrated a serious personality disorder. She had to be the decision-making partner and the stable factor in the partnership. While she was fit, well and working the family held together, aided by extended family support, and Sheila's warm and engaging personality. Her progressive illness, necessitating prolonged periods of hospitalisation, placed responsibilities on her husband which he found difficult, and then impossible, to cope with. Heavy drinking, irresponsible behaviour at work, bizarre demands became a regular pattern. When first diagnosed, Sheila had not wanted help – at that time admissions were not so frequent and she had the support of neighbours and extended family. The deaths of two key family members within two months of each other suddenly placed increased responsibility on Don, which he simply found impossible to cope with. Heavy drinking caused him to lose his job. Initially Sheila tried to cope in her customary way, using friends and neighbours, but the situation broke down during one of her admissions, when she finally sought help. A comprehensive network of help and support was established for her and her family, which freed Sheila from anxiety about her home situation, thus allowing her to benefit from hospitalisation and treatment. Supporting and sustaining Sheila was a crucial social work function. She recognised the source of her difficulties but felt trapped. While unable to change the basic fabric of her life and relationships, much was done to enable Sheila to function within it, thus improving the quality of her life.

Sheila was a tremendously courageous person who understood the nature of her illness and was able to think ahead and make plans to safeguard her small son's future upon her death. The framework established for Sheila and her family is illustrated in Figure 3.1 to demonstrate the degree of networking that can be necessary:

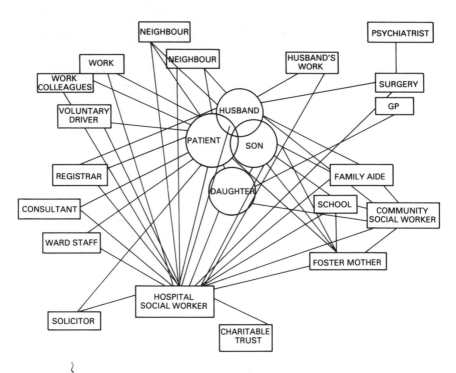

Figure 3.1.   Network of contacts and support for Sheila and family

In a hospital setting, situations of tragedy are not uncommon, where a social worker can only be 'reliably alongside.'

Case example: Luke was a young American medical student admitted to hospital, seriously injured after a road traffic accident. He was sightseeing with his sister and two other friends. The others had minor injuries. Luke's parents flew over – they were a close, kind, loving family. The social worker had been alerted to Luke's situation and that of his sister and friends early enough to have his parents met at the airport and driven to hospital. She arranged accommodation and maintained contact with them as they coped with a very worrying situation in a strange country, away from normal supports. The girls were assisted to return to the United States on their fixed return tickets – an extremely competent senior secretary in the social work department achieved this in liaison with a local travel agency sympathetic to the problem.

Luke improved and was transferred out of the intensive therapy unit. Negotiations were started to fly him home to the United States. At 8 p.m. Luke's parents bade him goodnight and returned to their accommodation. At 6 a.m. the next morning they were awakened by a security officer and rushed to the ward. Luke had died of a pulmonary embolism a few minutes earlier.

The social worker could do no more than be reliably alongside and help with practical matters in this time of tragedy for these parents. In situations like this, when defences are totally down and feelings uppermost, people reveal much of of themselves. The social worker is privileged to share so much at a time of great vulnerability and in return has to give much to form the bond that is essential for good social work. The art lies in remaining professional while being deeply touched.

Social workers can be the patient's single advocate and champion, sometimes even against family who, in anxiety, may want a 'safe' solution. In these situations the social worker will share in risk-taking with a mentally alert but physically frail, vulnerable elderly person who wants a final chance to return home despite the odds (see Chapter 9). The social worker's role here would be to support self-determination. Without her support this chance could be lost. Social workers should be ever mindful that people in hospital are vulnerable, not only because they face uncertainty, but also because they are out of their own environment and can feel out of control. They try to find out how people see their own problems and help them to make more rational decisions and choices at a time when their vision may be clouded. By giving patients time, by individualising them, by understanding their needs, patients are helped to retain their identity and maintain their resolve.

Patients do not only have emotional difficulties but also financial problems, even though they may receive some support from the state, and raising funds from charitable sources is still a necessity; to meet unexpectedly large heating bills, to buy driving lessons for a wife who the social worker knows will, in the fullness of time, be left a widow, to pay for a car service in order that the patient is enabled to hang on to her one independent activity – there are many other constructive and creative ways in which these funds can be used to ease the burden of long-term and chronic ill health, thus assisting the healing process.

Helping people to cope with their crisis is clearly a vital part of the social worker's task in hospital, but with the development of medical technology and treatment, people who had previously succumbed to their illness, or at best had to remain in institutional care, now survive and are able to consider returning home or live in the community with appropriate support networks. Support systems have developed in keeping with this need and social workers in hospital are important coordinators in the assessment process, linking the hospital with the community. (see Figure 3.1) Other support systems, created by the local authority, as opposed to private and family ones as used for Sheila, are home help, day care, etc. These are vital services. While the aim is the discharge of the patient from hospital, the social worker's involvement ensures that the discharge is appropriate, free from unnecessary anxiety, in the best interest of the patient and that all available help and support has been considered. It is an important function in the all-round well-being of the patient and has therapeutic value.

Hospital social workers should be aware of the psycho/social implications, the impact of the illness, disability or loss, and take a holistic approach. Where necessary they are proactive, anticipating needs and reactions and 'reaching out' to patients. They have a professional responsibility to be familiar with local services and resources and should be imaginative in their use of them. They also have a responsibility and duty to influence their co-professionals and the institution in which they work to ensure that the medical and surgical expertise offered is balanced by an awareness of the patients' social and personal needs, thus completing the healing process.

3.2 Why hospital-based?

Every hospital, unit or ward has its own culture. To be effective the social worker needs to be part of that culture, understand how it functions and know its norms and etiquette. Medics can be quite rigid about matters of etiquette; e.g. who refers what to whom. Each profession has its own historically laid-down rules and responsibilities. For example, the ward sister is in charge of the ward, has responsibility for it; it is therefore important for the social worker to catch her eye when entering a ward, to make sure the sister knows that she is not interfering with the good running of the ward. This is a matter of common politeness, and important in maintaining good relationships. Social workers should try to know and understand the rules, responsibilities and etiquette of all the professions present in the institution, so that they can either work within those rules and avoid giving offence, or, when the rules have to be broken, it is done knowingly, in a tactful manner, and for a good reason: in the patient's best interest.

Differing medical situations give rise to different sets of medical or psycho-social problems and needs. These have to be identified and understood if appropriate and timely help is to be offered. Thus, in a hospital with multiple units or several specialist units, hospital social workers have to be unit attached if they hope to identify the medico/psycho-social needs of the patients and understand the unit, how it functions and 'who does what and when'. Unit attachment allows for the accumulation of a body of knowledge relevant to the particular medical condition and the set of problems it creates for the patient. This body of knowledge leads to the development of expertise crucial to good medical social work practice. Expertise is essential if one is to be credible. Credibility leads to trust, trust to acceptability. In a setting where there is an emphasis on speciality and expertise it need hardly be said that credibility is not easily gained. It is essential that social workers in this setting speak with confidence based on experience and with authority on their subject.

Being part of a unit and thus part of the treatment team – which will be discussed later in this chapter – allows the social worker to target her help in conjunction with the rest of the team. She is able to contribute to team thinking in terms of plans and treatment programme, giving the team the benefit of her knowledge of the family dynamics, the social situation and the psycho-social needs of the patient where this is relevant, and of the close connection between physical, social and emotional functioning. The social worker's traditional holistic approach will encourage the team to view the patient as part of the constellation of his family and environment rather than as an isolated entity. Interpretation of the patient's or family's needs is important and the social worker is in the best position to put this across if she is a credible and an effective member of the treatment team.

Where social workers have abandoned unit attachment, working an allocation system, they may function as good social workers but they are less effective as *medical* social workers. Without the knowledge base of the implications of particular medical situations, without team membership, much is lost to the patient whose interest should be their primary concern.

3.3 How hospital social workers work

Hospital patients come from a wide spectrum of society. Most will never have had contact with social workers and will be puzzled at first by the suggestion that a social worker see them, associating social workers either with welfare benefits and therefore concerned with the poor and needy or simply 'the welfare' to do with people who need help to manage their affairs. Few will know that social workers deal with feelings, and even less that social workers are concerned with reactions to loss. There is, therefore a need for the social worker to reach out and, having reached out, they find that people who are vulnerable respond very quickly to interest and understanding.

Interviewing in a ward, whether there is one other person or three, is a skill social workers have to develop very early in their careers – the skill to create an oasis, space, 'bubble' of confidentiality, an environment of safety and trust (in a busy, often noisy atmosphere) within which the patient can react; to convey to her that she is worthy of attention. The social worker has to convey caring, concern, genuine warmth and, using body language, help the patient relax and believe that time is hers (despite the many other pressing demands in the background of the worker's mind). She has to empathise while also assessing, leaping ahead in her mind with plans which have to be tentatively made in readiness to discuss with the patient at a later stage, when she is emotionally receptive. This last however, can be a problem, as patients do not stay in hospital for very long. Hospital social workers have to be experts at creating this space, and getting the patient's trust as fast as their physical condition allows, or they will find that the patient has been discharged before the process is complete.

Social work in a hospital involves a great deal of liaison both with co-professionals within the hospital and with services and agencies outside. Social workers need to be experts at networking. To be effective as the patient's advocate as well as an advocate for their profession, they need to be articulate orally and on paper. Advocacy touches upon the educational aspects of their work and the influence they have upon the institution in which they work. In teaching hospitals, with the constant movement of junior medical staff – the future consultants – this is a vital and very necessary part of their function. The educational process encompasses the need to alert team colleagues to potential problems – helping them to identify vulnerable patients, making them aware of psycho-social reactions and needs.

The hospital social worker works best and most effectively if she is both personally and professionally secure. She has to be able to stand up to scrutiny and value her professional contribution. She has to have the ability to communicate well, formally and informally, with hospital staff and with agencies outside. She has to be tactful and be aware of the sensibilities of team members, respecting them for their particular skills when sharing patient care. They must be comfortable working with a wide range of social classes – normally coping and capable people who will be relating to social workers for the first time as they work towards 'new equilibriums'. She must be able to work with, and stay with, emotional pain, and be reliable and consistent in her relationship with patients whose world can be changing around them.

3.4 Influence and impact on the institution

The presence of hospital social workers has a positive impact on the institution if they function and operate from a firm knowledge base and are perceived to be part of that institution, subject to the same pressures and stresses. They cannot easily influence or hope to influence change from afar. Social workers need to know the people who work within the institution, understand how it functions and identify the system(s) which need modification or change. They are a small group of professionals, outnumbered by medical and nursing colleagues. To be heard, social workers must speak with clear voices and with authority based on experience and knowledge. Knowing key people, where the power lies in the many different departments, and how the relevant people think and function is crucial – a unit attachment system allows individual social workers this opportunity on a small scale – the line manager has to have the overall picture.

Influence can be subtle but have far-reaching effects on the quality of service to the patients. Social workers have a responsibility to be advocates for patients wherever this is indicated. Influence begins on a day-to-day working basis where there is opportunity to 'educate' and sensitise co-professionals to the patients' emotional and personal needs. An in-depth knowledge of a unit allows the social worker to suggest improvements to existing systems or the introduction of new systems with the full understanding and co-operation of other staff, essential if the changes are to become a recognised part of the hospital service.

Examples of change:

1. A social worker's recognition of the needs of patients following amputation, after working on a unit for six months, led to the development of a proactive comprehensive programme of care which took account of their

psycho-social and rehabilitation needs. Once made aware, the consultant concerned became a powerful advocate, active on a steering committee where representatives from the hospital team, rehabilitation centre and community met to discuss the relevant issues for the first time. The result was a much improved service, which patients valued and responded to.

2. A social worker's recognition of the special needs of women facing breast surgery, particularly at the time of diagnosis, and arranging, with the co-operation of out-patient clinic staff, to be visibly present in the out-patients' department led to this becoming a recognised part of the service in the hospital where the social worker is available to support the patient at a time of shock and emotional turmoil.

3. Alerting intensive therapy unit staff to the special needs of out of town/country patients and relatives, who must cope with heightened emotions in strange surroundings and without their normal framework of support, led to patients and relatives being brought to the attention of the social work department so that help could be offered, as in the case of Luke's family.

4. Social assessment, presence at weekly ward meetings, ward rounds and social reporting, all serve to remind co-professionals of the psycho-social elements of illness.

This work is both demanding and very satisfying – the setting allows social workers to be creative and imaginative. They are in the privileged position of being in situations of crisis when help, given at the right time, can have a positive outcome.

It is not reality that makes cowards of people but dreams, nightmares, not nice dreams. If one can remove the nightmare quality, and at the same time help them face reality, people really have a tremendous resistance and a tremendous amount of strength.

3.5 *Working with other professions: The multidisciplinary team*

The 1974 report *Social Work Support for the Health Service* stated:

We suggest that teamwork in a clinical situation means that all members of the team accept that each has a professional contribution to make in his own right; and that it is both the right, and equally, the responsibility of each member of the team to make that contribution if the patient needs it. Such a responsibility derives not from the prescription of the head of the team, but from the right of the patient to have the benefit of all the team's skills as he needs them.

It is a paradox in hospital work that the social worker's closest colleagues, the people with whom she is working on a daily, even hourly basis, are employed by a different authority, i.e. the health authority as opposed to the local authority (county council, metropolitan borough or Scottish region). This can at times become a problem, particularly if there is an element of conflict between the two authorities, but, that said, we shall now look in some detail at day-to-day working relationships, and the implications of being a member of a multidisciplinary team.

3.5.1 The environment

In order to achieve effective working relationships, the social worker needs a sound knowledge base of her own and her colleagues' work. As has been emphasised earlier she will be working with highly trained and articulate people, and needs to be able to combine an understanding of the implications of the medical situation with an ability to present the social work perspective despite sometimes feeling a lone voice in discussion. She cannot work in isolation from other staff, and disasters in terms of patient care and interdisciplinary relationships will result if she tries to. This means that the social worker is operating in a very complex environment, working at the very least with many nursing and medical staff, and often with physiotherapist, occupational therapist, dietitian, speech therapist, psychologist, etc. as well. The need for a cohesive team, which can work towards joint decisions and collective care for patients becomes very clear, as is the need for staff to share a basic philosophy in their attitudes towards the care and treatment of the patient.

The social worker has to remember that the patient initially came to the hospital for diagnosis and/or treatment, and to be highly sensitive to her needs *as* a sick person. For example, a worker who disturbs patients' meal-times or rest times to talk, or is unaware of their needs for say, a commode, or pain relief, is helping neither the patient nor her own credibility on the ward. She must also be sensitive to the fact that the patient is tied to his bed and cannot walk out on an interview when he would have liked to do so. Most patients are referred by other staff, have not themselves asked for social work help, or may be too polite to tell the worker to go. Hospital social workers have therefore to be specially aware of what the person who is being interviewed tells them by his or her body language and/or silences and other reactions.

3.5.2 Working relationships

The development of any close working relationship will depend partly on the congruence of the stated aims of the group, and partly on the more subtle interplay of personalities, and the degree to which mutual respect, sensitivity and interest can be built up. All staff are operating under increasing pressure, as financial restraints continue to bite, and to understand each other's pressures rather than being preoccupied with one's own, can only help relationships. Most people are comforted and heartened by hearing a colleague say: 'I *couldn't* do your job!' It will help working relationships enormously if the social worker understands the routine of the ward, and the pressures of the particularly busy times, and conversely, if the ward staff understand some of the pressures on the social worker and that, for example, if a home visit from the ward has been planned for 2 p.m., it is important that the patient is ready and not still deeply asleep at that time.

It is stating the obvious to say that the boundaries between the different professionals are usually clear, but there can be significant areas of overlap. Who, for example, should see a patient's relative to discuss care after hospitalisation? Who should talk with the patient about her anxieties concerning her diagnosis? Doctors, nurses and social workers may all do this, but clearly they should undertake it in a planned, cohesive way, rather than duplicate their labour and irritate patients and relatives by repeated and uncoordinated approaches. Equally, is it the task of the social worker to encourage a reluctant patient to take fluids or mobilise, or even to hold a bowl while the patient who is being interviewed is sick? Opinions will vary! Opinions will also vary as to whether the social worker should answer the ward telephone if all the nurses are invisible attending to patients, and whether it is an inappropriate use of time to help a nurse make a bed when she then wants the nurse's attention for discussing a patient. The key point is that there can be overlaps of function alongside clearly differentiated tasks: these need to be carefully handled so that they enhance working relationships and the service to the patient, and do not result in the misunderstandings and resentments which can occur all too easily when people are working under pressure.

3.5.3 Communication

One essential thread which runs through the whole field of interdisciplinary working relationships is communication. It is easy to agree that this is vital, but it can be quite difficult to achieve in a fast-moving and highly complex environment. The information to be communicated will normally, at its most basic, be the request from a member of staff to the social worker to see a patient, and the feed-back from the social worker to the medical and nursing staff. Commonly however, discussion will take place even at the point of referral – how long will the patient be in hospital, what do ward staff know about the family background? Then there will often be continued discussion, feed-back and joint planning as the situation progresses. Perhaps the patient is recovering less well than had been anticipated – how will she and her family react to this? Or perhaps a huge family row took place last night, when the social worker was off duty. All staff need to keep up to date with the patient's situation so that their input remains relevant and effective.

Methods of communication vary from the formal to the very informal, from ward round and ward meetings led by senior medical staff to chats in the corridor, and are both oral and written. A weekly formalised discussion will have the advantage that most team members will be present, so joint discussion and planning can take place. A week however is a long time in a hospital, and new facts can emerge every day, so there needs to be a continuous interchange of information. Much of this will be by word of mouth, but in view of the many different members of staff involved there is often a case to be made for the social worker to write in the medical and nursing records, so that what has, or has not, been achieved is quite clear to all. At the same time the worker has to take care never to include information the patient has expressly designated as confidential. Although in most hospitals social workers are free to consult medical notes and add their own to them, social work records belong to the employing authority, and are not available to other hospital staff. Confidential information should be confined to them. Informal methods of communication tend to have a friendly feel to them, but more formal or written information is more enduring. Both therefore have their place and both should be used.

3.5.4 Medical knowledge

As hospital-based social workers are working with patients who are ill or disabled, and undergoing diagnosis and treatment, it is evident that the greater the extent of their medical knowledge, the greater will be their ability to offer appropriate help. In the past, when there was a separate training for each branch of social work, the medical social work courses contained a large input of basic anatomy and physiology, and teaching about a number of medical specialities. This is almost wholly lacking in generic social work courses, and many social workers have to fall back on what they learned at school or have picked up subsequently, combined – and this is very important – with learning on the job. This can be through reading a textbook at the appropriate level, and by asking the medical, nursing and other staff they work with, for explanations, which are usually willingly given. It is however incumbent on social workers to become familiar as quickly as possible with the medical conditions which will be met with in the unit in which they work, in order to understand what it means to the patient to have for example an ileostomy, or hemiplegia, and the implications of the diagnosis for his family.

Medical knowledge does however appear to be infinite, and is constantly increasing. Most social workers will feel that there is some knowledge they do not require, such as perhaps the understanding of a patient's biochemical values, but many will feel that great satisfaction and increased integration with their units can be gained by the extending of their medical knowledge and an ability to ask informative questions can only result in a better service to clients.

3.6 Working with area-based social work colleagues

Since 1974 hospital social workers have been employed by local authorities rather than health authorities. They therefore share the same employer as nearly all area social workers, and for many years have had a common generic training, so one would anticipate that working relationships would be close, trusting and creative. Hospital social workers do however work in a very different environment which has different perspectives and pressures, and as with any group, particularly perhaps between those who work inside an institution and those who work outside, myths and fantasies can abound, and the situation can lend itself to scapegoating. This process is not of course confined to social workers – one has only to hear hospital doctors and general practitioners, or ward nurses and community (district) nurses complaining about each other to realise this, but where there is a structure which lends itself to problems and misunderstandings a lot of work will be required to overcome them. It is of course hard for people who work in widely differing settings and yet who at times have to work closely together to understand each other's problems, particularly if the problem is experienced solely by one group and is far outside the experience of the others. Furthermore, the taxing workloads of most social workers, and others such as home care organisers, can mean, understandably, that it is hard to recognise each other's problems, and they prefer to think that the other could provide a solution if only they would 'co-operate'. This however is not the path to closer working relationships.

3.6.1 Impact of geographical distance

By definition, area-based social workers will usually work within a defined geographical territory, whether this is called a division, area, locality, etc., though of course in a rural area the territory to be covered will be very much larger than within a city. A hospital by contrast only occasionally takes its patients on a fixed geographical basis: in general the larger the hospital, the wider the area from which it will take patients, and highly specialised and teaching hospitals can accept patients not only from all over the country, but even from overseas. All these patients are potential clients for the social workers. Health authorities are sometimes co-terminous with county boundaries, but regional health authorities will normally cover several counties, so at the very least a hospital social worker will be working with staff in divisional offices across the county, and sometimes in neighbouring counties. One small district general hospital, for instance, is situated only just inside the boundary of its own county and receives a large number of patients from three neighbouring counties: the social workers based in that hospital have to develop equally close working relationships with colleagues in these three counties as with their fellow employees in their own county. By contrast however there are the small community hospitals (often formerly called cottage hospitals), whose patients remain under their general practitioners: they may have the part-time service of a social worker who is based either in the local area team, or within the hospital social work structure, but in either case she will be working with perhaps only one or two social work offices and can therefore form much closer links with colleagues there.

In general, the wide geographical areas covered involve hospital social workers in building relationships over the telephone, but close links can be formed and then it becomes a great pleasure to meet the person who has been a telephone contact over many months. Another problem is that, even within the same authority, procedures may vary slightly from one local office to the next, and the hospital social worker needs to become familiar with these variations in order to use the services appropriately. This is hardest when there is a change in organisation and familiar landmarks disappear: who do we now send the application to for a telephone? At all costs however, the 'Dear Sir/Madam'-type communication should be avoided in one's own authority, as it sounds very impersonal and bureaucratic and leads to increased feelings of distance between different officers and departments.

3.6.2 Working together

The overriding aim should be to achieve what is in the best interests of the client/patient, as well as what is practicable for the social workers concerned. Before looking at true joint working, some attention should be given to the sometimes thorny area of referrals from one group to the other, into and out of hospital social work departments. There are basically three variables to be weighed up: (a) how far there is a medical component to the social problem, (b) the distance from the hospital, and (c) the priorities of the social workers concerned. A client whose problems stem from a complex and continuing illness or disability is more likely to be the continued responsibility of the hospital social worker, whereas one whose problems are essentially family centred, even though they come to light in the course of an admission to hospital, may more appropriately be the responsibility of the area team social worker. The question of the priorities of the different teams can be a problem however, particularly when all are feeling hard pressed by volume of work. Ill, disabled and elderly people tend to be a low priority for generic teams struggling with unallocated child abuse cases, on the other hand hospital teams cannot provide a continuing service for the myriads of people, out-patients as well as in-patients, who pass through the hospital doors.

It can happen that a community social worker already knows a client before she is admitted to hospital. It is immensely helpful if that social worker can let the hospital team know, partly to avoid confusion if the client is independently referred to the hospital social worker, and partly so that a coherent way of working together can be planned. Depending on the nature of the problem, and the relationship the social worker already has with the client, she may want to continue to work closely with her while in hospital, sometimes using her hospital colleague as an information resource or to facilitate communication with ward staff. Equally it may be decided that it is in the client's interest for the hospital social worker to be the key worker, particularly for example at a time of crisis when she might need to be visited daily, or where close collaboration with other hospital staff is essential.

As when working closely with colleagues from other disciplines, the ability to work with a social worker from another setting can be extremely satisfying. Each can be a mine of information for the other, relationships are built up, and it can feel a comfort to be working with a colleague in a very complex case. There can of course also be conflict, in the absence of procedures defining every situation; for example should it be the local area team or the hospital team who arrange care for the dependent relative (whether child, elderly or mentally handicapped) of a patient who has to come into hospital as an emergency? There can be some hard negotiation in these grey areas, but equally, when one member of the local intake team says, 'Well, you did the last, so we will do this one', it indicates a good working relationship.

It will be clear that a hospital is a complex place in which to work, with the number of different professionals, each with their own priorities and philosophy with whom the worker has to build a working relationship, its organisational complexities, which have to become familiar and in which crisis and loss have to be faced by patients and their families. As in most other areas of human endeavour, relationships particularly with so wide a range of co-professionals, will not always be smooth, and there can be considerable differences of perspective alongside a fundamental commitment to the welfare of those in need. The social worker cannot function in isolation and must not only be able to work closely with other colleagues both within and outside the institution, but must be sufficiently skilled and secure in her competence to give an effective service to people who are facing personal tragedy.

Notes

1. Caplan, Gerald, *Crisis Intervention*, New York: Family Service Association of America, 1966.

Suggestions for further reading

Bartlett, Harriett M., *Some Aspects of Social Casework in a Medical Setting*, Chicago: American Association of Medical Social Workers, 1940.

Butrym, Zofia, *Social Work in Medical Care*, London: Routledge & Kegan Paul, 1967.

Downie, R. S., and Telfer, E. *Caring and Curing: A Philosophy of Medicine and Social Work*, London: Methuen, 1980.

Germain, C.B., *Social Work Practice in Health Care*, New York: Free Press, 1984.

Law, Elizabeth, *A Study of Patterns of Work and Use of Time*, City of Manchester Social Services Department, 1976 (enquiries to Mrs E. Law, Manchester Social Services Department).

CHAPTER 4

Psychological problems in chronic illness

JULIET AUER

This chapter focuses on the psychological problems experienced in severe, disabling physical conditions and the handicaps they present. Disability is here defined as a loss or reduction of functional ability,[1] while handicap is the disadvantage or restriction of activity caused by disability. Handicap therefore arises from the interaction of disability with social and environmental conditions. The material is largely drawn from work with patients in chronic renal failure, maintained on dialysis. Milder chronic complaints can cause either less marked, or similar problems, according to the way in which they are perceived by the patient and interact to produce handicap. Epilepsy, for example, may cause very little disability, but is potentially handicapping, due to social stigma and limitations in educational opportunity and choice of job. It would make little difference to a writer, but would drastically affect a professional driver, pilot or scaffolder. This chapter does not specifically address the very large topic of chronic mental illness, but this area shares much in common with chronic physical illness, particularly in the problems of stigma leading to social isolation,[2] financial disadvantage[3] and changes in ability to cope with everyday life. The families of sufferers, who are involved in care, and professional staff involved in treatment, are subject to long-term stresses in both physical and mental illness. At the outset it is necessary to define chronic illness, and the ways in which it differs from acute illness, in order to appreciate the nature of work with the chronically ill patient.

4.1 Differences between acute and chronic illness

In general terms, acute illness is a temporary interruption in the normal pattern of living, following which there is a return to previous health. Chronic illness involves permanent changes and adjustments in living, because the patient can never fully recover, and is likely to deteriorate rather than improve over time. These are the extreme ends of what is in reality a continuum. Many conditions are relapsing, fluctuating or intermittent, causing specific stresses due to the frequent change in circumstances. Other acute admissions, for example termination of pregnancy or hysterectomy, may have a deep psychological significance to the patient, leading to the need for counselling and adjustment.

In addition to the objective severity of the illness, there is the contribution of attitude and state of mind, which can have immense influence on perceived disability and actual rehabilitation. All conditions, whether acute, chronic or fluctuating, benefit from sensitive help, aimed at using the patient's internal resources and external supports to achieve the best and fullest life that is possible.

4.2 Acute illness

4.2.1 Patient attitudes in acute illness

The patient entering hospital with an acute condition, for example cholecystitis, or the need for hysterectomy, may have been well throughout life, spend ten days in hospital for an operation, and remain well thereafter. In such a case, it is usually of little long-term importance to the patient whether good relationships are formed with the hospital staff, because there will be no need to sustain a long-term interaction. The chief concern is whether the operation is performed competently, and the medical and nursing care lead to a swift and uncomplicated recovery. If there are dissatisfactions the patient may feel free to complain, even at the risk of being labelled as difficult. There may be pain, fear of medical procedures, fear of what may be discovered during investigations, difficulty in sleeping, loss of privacy, dislike of hospital food or rules, but there is also an awareness of the temporary nature of the role as patient. This is not the real world, but a short ordeal, which will recede from the memory on returning to the safe and familiar. He or she is free to enjoy some aspects of the situation, such as the sympathy and concern of family and friends, the attention, and the injunctions to take it easy. There should be no threat to work status and no serious change in family relationships or finances due to the illness. Soon there will be a resumption of previous patterns, interests, hobbies and social life. As a result the individual's sense of identity is not threatened.

4.2.2 Attitudes of others to acute illness

When an illness is time-limited, family, friends, employers and even creditors are able to rise to the occasion with reserves of goodwill. They are aware that the patient will be fit to return to normal roles at work and as husband/father or wife/mother after this short episode. Temporary responsibility for the partner's role is within the capacity of most spouses, and is often willingly embraced in the short term. Spouse and family will probably experience anxiety, because the very fact of hospital admission has worrying associations. The hospital is an alien environment, in which others are in control. Once uncertainty over the outcome is over and recovery starts, the anxiety is largely dissipated in relief and gratitude.

In acute illness, the patient is permitted to adopt a sick role, and encouraged, by medical professionals, family and employers, to indulge this in order to facilitate a return to health. Once home, there is a mandatory period of convalescence, the visits of friends and relatives, ('Not too long just at first') and the jokes about some people being willing to go through anything to get a holiday. Everybody is aware that the worst is over. The whole episode follows an unwritten, ritualistic procedure, in which all participants know not only the rules, but even the script. Even death and bereavement, although deeply distressing, have acknowledged frameworks of behaviour within which people are able to respond appropriately. Many cultures and faiths have defined a time scale for the stages of mourning, to assist all concerned in the proper expression of feelings.

Acute illness is largely managed on an in-patient basis, with little medical follow-up after discharge from hospital. In spite of this, there is an important role for the social worker, since any admission to hospital can be a crisis for patient and family, especially if it is an emergency admission. There are not only practical problems such as care of dependents and payment of bills, but also psychological considerations. The unaccustomed vulnerability of the patient may trigger the release of pent-up emotions, or regressed behaviour that are frightening in their intensity. It is also well documented that certain events and injuries, whether medically severe or not, can lead to long- term psychological problems, especially if accompanied by shock, or a threat to the integrity of the personality. Post traumatic stress disorder is now well recognised and is less likely to be diagnosed as malingering. Crisis counselling may therefore be of great importance.

4.3 Chronic illness

At the other end of the scale is the patient who is diagnosed as having a chronic condition. Whether this is comparatively mild, or serious and life threatening, the implications are quite different from those of acute illness. This is a case of learning to live with illness, and trying to ignore or accommodate symptoms. Discharge from hospital represents not the start of a return to normality, but of discovering limitations which will probably increase with time.

4.3.1 Attitudes in chronic illness

In chronic illness, work, leisure, relationships, marital roles, finances, housing and social life may all be threatened. The consequences for partners and families are no less far reaching. The self-esteem and identity of the patients are severely threatened by the diagnosis. For most sufferers there can be no gratification from expressions of sympathy or offers of help, (even if the patient feels grateful), because the situation has become permanently unequal, with the patient at a disadvantage. Sympathy has subtly changed into pity from the patient's viewpoint, thereby emphasising a new and inadequate status. In contrast with acute illness, there is a very real sense in which people do not know what to say. There is no script or prescribed ritual for either patient, family or others. This can make contact with patient and family uncomfortable, or even socially embarrassing, which can lead to withdrawal and avoidance. Ironically, the adoption of a sick role is not encouraged, but the behaviour of others gives the message that the patient is now different. The object, following diagnosis, is not to take it easy and get back to normal, but to attack the hard task of learning to accept a changed situation as the future normality. The world of doctors, hospitals, illness and treatment are to be the reality, and full health the receding memory. Many feel so different and set apart, that they find it hard to regain a sense of belonging in the normal world. The result is a degree of social isolation.

Perhaps for this reason there is an increased bond with others in the same situation, and with health care professionals. At first, doctors and nurses assume great importance to the patient, because they have become invested with long-term power and influence over the future. They therefore need to be pleased and placated, by means of being a good patient, just as one needed to please and placate parents by being a good child. This does not necessarily mean that all the rules are obeyed, but that a patient does not want to be caught breaking them, and incur displeasure. Many treatment procedures can be performed with gentleness and consideration, or with less of these characteristics. The good patient, who is cheerful and uncomplaining, is more likely to be treated well.

Whether consciously or unconsciously, most patients experience these attitudes, at least in the first few months. In many they are shown overtly. Others respond to the same beliefs with resentment, truculence and rebellion, which is another manifestation of the same regressed attitude to those with presumed or actual authority and power. Since neither attitude is healthy, most good units dealing with chronic conditions try to establish a more adult and equal relationship. Unfortunately, human nature being as it is, the patient who tries to please is usually less trouble, and therefore genuinely more acceptable to staff than the rebel, (with the exception of the 'charming rogue' for whom all seem to have a sneaking affection). As a result, the dependent attitude tends to be reinforced. Over time, a more realistic view tends to emerge, in which unit staff are accepted as human beings rather than stereotypes.

Real relationships are then possible, and may grow into firm friendships. Many chronically sick patients come to regard the hospital unit they attend as a second home, and the permanent staff as a second family.

4.3.2 Implications for social work practice

In order to help in treatment planning, the social worker will need to get to know the patient, and those who will be affected by the change of circumstances. An initial social report may be requested by the medical staff, and used to decide what treatment regimes will be possible and convenient. Chronic illness is largely managed on an out-patient basis, so a pre-discharge home visit with the patient is extremely helpful in order to assess possible future problems. It is preferable to talk to everyone involved on their own territory, since a more natural response can be obtained than in the hospital surroundings. It is important to see family dynamics in operation, to get an early impression of the coping mechanisms that are habitually used, and any particular family stresses. Certain strengths and weaknesses in the patient's situation may be immediately apparent.

Patient and family are usually eager to discuss information they have already received from medical and nursing staff, and to ask questions. Evidence to a CCETSW working party (1974) shows that patients expect the Social Worker to be 'knowledgeable about the nature, process and characteristics of handicapping conditions and their effects on them and their families.[4] This permits the social worker to find out how much has been heard, how much understood, and the attitudes of the family to the illness. Myths and misconceptions about the disease and its treatment can be addressed. A common fear is that the illness may be hereditary. If this is not the case, reassurance can be given. If the fear is well grounded, medical advice and/or genetic counselling can be arranged.

The home visit will also give an insight into the patient's interests and hobbies, which are often evident in family photographs, books, or a well tended garden. Enquiries into work, interests and social life will enable a quick assessment of the degree of change and adjustment that the patient is likely to face over the coming months or years. Any mobility problems, or potential hazards in the home can be noted for referral to the occupational therapist, who may be able to attend at the same time. Available space for treatment equipment, such as oxygen cylinders for chronic obstructive airways disease, lifts or hoists for patients with neurological damage and wheelchair access, needs consideration. Since rehousing may be needed, either urgently or in the future, due to an expected deterioration in mobility or independence, an early visit will enable applications to proceed as quickly as possible. The need for Attendance or Mobility Allowance can also be judged and acted upon. If care problems are anticipated, a visit from the home care organiser and district nurse will be planned.

Initially a practical focus is most reassuring to the patient and family. This will lay foundations for a trusting relationship in which emotional problems can also be discussed. These may be evident from the start, but timing is important. To try to face the patient, or partner, with delicate issues without invitation is destructive to the therapeutic relationship. The invitation is sometimes direct, but more usually oblique. It may be expressed in body language or a hesitation, but it needs to be accurately read. The social worker should therefore be able to converse in a relaxed way, while maintaining acute observation and sensitivity to expression, gesture and omissions from others.

In most cases, the patient will be attending hospital again, as an in- or out-patient, at frequent intervals. In this case it is not necessary or desirable to make a formal appointment, but it is important, for the development of a long-term relationship, that the social worker should be visible and accessible in clinic and ward, and to greet the patient by name. In a large and impersonal hospital, this seems to carry great significance for those who feel that they are entering an institutional world. If one is also able to remember the names of family members or pets, and ask after them, it is even better. Most of the hospital staff will not have seen the patient at home. The visit makes the social worker into a reassuring link between the two worlds, who will almost certainly be told, directly or indirectly, if there are any problems. It is necessary to establish from the start, that confidentiality will be maintained, unless permission is given for information to be shared with the other members of the multidisciplinary team.

In cases of chronic illness there is usually some immediate practical financial or crisis-based work to be done, but the main objective, which needs to be borne in mind from the start, is to establish a relationship with long-term therapeutic potential.

4.4 Reactions of patients to diagnosis of chronic illness

The first reaction to the diagnosis of a severe chronic condition, such as multiple sclerosis, Parkinson's disease, or chronic renal failure, is often shock or disbelief. This is usually followed by a degree of anger and self-pity, summed up in the question 'Why me?'. This is often expanded to 'Why now?', since, whenever the diagnosis is made, it is seen as being at the worst possible time, whether this is when a young adult is beginning to create an independent life, or at the start of marriage, or before the children are grown up, or at the peak of one's career, or, indeed, when the patient has just retired and has time to enjoy the freedom and leisure which should follow a lifetime's work.

There is also an attempt to find reasons, or apportion blame. It is not easy for people to accept that there is no reason, and no one to blame for what has happened. It is more comfortable to have a rationale, or to direct anger at a person or situation, (even at oneself), than to accept that fate, God, or bad luck has singled one out for cruel treatment. It is human nature to want life to be both logical, fair and under one's control. A further reaction which is often present is a paradoxical relief. Many chronic illnesses, in particular degenerative diseases of the nervous system such as multiple sclerosis, are diagnosed following years of transient or ill-defined symptoms, which may have puzzled the medical profession. Tests may have been inconclusive and the patient told that the problem could be psychosomatic. Patients with renal failure often fear that they have cancer, because of weight loss, lack of energy and pallor. The positive diagnosis, even if unwelcome, ends uncertainty and explains vague symptoms that could have been due to something worse. It also justifies the patient's feeling that there was something wrong other than a guilt-provoking inability to cope. It is not surprising that in this initial state of turmoil, the patient is often unwilling, or unable to address the future.

A surprising number of patients choose this moment to

complete unfinished business, often from the distant past. Some wish to grieve for a baby lost at birth, or a parent's death. Others wish to marry a longstanding co-habitee and legitimise children. The crisis of the diagnosis, especially if potentially life-threatening, seems to focus the mind on putting the past to rights. Only when this is complete can progress occur.[5]

The next stage, which may be reached in days, or take months, is the first attempt to look forward. Three common reactions deserve mention. The first is an *unrealistic optimism*, based on a buoyant determination that the illness and treatment are not to be allowed to change anything. The patient clings to the conviction that all that is needed is willpower and courage, or that the implications of the diagnosis are not severe, or even that the diagnosis was incorrect. This attitude has much to recommend it, but often gives way to depression and despair when the full impact of the limitations and necessary adjustments to life begin to impinge. It is a dysfunctional use of denial, that is bound to collide painfully with reality before long. A second coping response is to look for hope and relief, even cure, from *alternative medicine*. This may involve herbal medicines, diets, meditation, psychic healing, acupuncture, reflexology or simple faith. If pursued in conjunction with conventional medicine, the outcome is almost always beneficial, since a positive attitude and high morale cannot be overestimated as factors mitigating chronic illness, but patients who substitute alternative therapies, or pin their hope on a miracle cure, are brought up against reality sooner or later, with or without actual risk or damage due to rejecting conventional therapy. There is then the need to start a realistic adjustment all over again, following disillusionment. These two reactions are, nevertheless, positive and active. The third response is one of *passive compliance and resignation*. All responsibility is delegated to the doctors, nurses and paramedical staff, because the patient feels helpless, and is happy to leave everything to the experts. This attitude may be appropriate in acute illness, but is unlikely to lead to a good adjustment in chronic conditions, where an active partnership with medical professionals, and a healthy degree of defiance and denial offer the best adjustment. This of course takes time. As an early response, passivity is harmless and natural, but independence and 'fight' need to be gently fostered if they do not grow naturally.

Periods of over-optimism and of depression are usual in the early stages of chronic illness, but, for most, settle into adjustment in the course of time. The social worker can facilitate this process of adjustment through a number of practical and psychological interventions. The following case demonstrates how great the overlap between the two can be, and how a seemingly trivial incident can be used to the patient's advantage.

Case example: A middle-aged divorcee, with recently diagnosed renal failure treated by continuous peritoneal dialysis, felt ugly and out of control of her life. She was an attractive and highly fastidious woman, who felt disfigured by the abdominal peritoneal dialysis catheter, and was very depressed. She had moved house just before starting treatment, to a pretty flat in a new housing development. Arranging a home visit over the phone, the social worker was told she would recognise the flat because it was the only one with a large pile of dirty empty boxes outside the front door. They had been used to transport small items during the move. In the course of the visit, the woman described all her problems as overwhelming. Her whole life was a mess, and not worth living. It was very apparent from the beautifully kept house, and the woman herself, who was well dressed and made up, that her self-esteem was at least partially intact. Inside the house, everything was in order. What she presented to the outside world was the heap of dirty boxes. It was too expensive, she said, to get someone to take them away, and she hadn't the energy. They had been there for weeks, and would have to stay. Faced with such overt two-level, or symbolic communication, it is important to respond constructively and in a like manner. On leaving, the social worker therefore said that she could put a number of them into the boot of her car and dispose of them. The woman enthusiastically helped the social worker to load them. The social worker was careful to pack-in most, but not all the boxes, and apologised for not being able to get rid of the problem. The woman was delighted. She said that she could easily get the remaining few boxes into her own car, and take them to the dump. (Her car, which was standing outside, was rather larger than the social worker's, and would certainly have accommodated the whole pile). To have removed *all* the rubbish, which was in some way representing her negative feelings about herself, could have reinforced her feelings of being unable to help herself. To reduce it to a level she felt competent to handle, enabled her to take a positive step towards increasing her self esteem. Two days later she had cleared the boxes and made the front of the house attractive.

4.5 Attitudes and problems within the family

The suffering of the spouse and family of the patient are often underestimated, and need special consideration, especially by the social worker. Patients who are chronically sick are seldom easy people to live with, since much of their emotional and physical energy is absorbed in coping with the illness and their own feelings. Those who feel less than well are often withdrawn and uncommunicative. This may be rationalised as 'not wanting to worry others', but succeeds in creating more distress than it saves. The spouse can often do no right. If he or she shows frequent concern, it is rebuffed as 'fussing'. If no concern is expressed, the spouse is accused of not caring.

4.5.1 Irritability

This is one of the most frequent psychological problems of chronic illness, due to frustration, depression, fatigue or worry. It is commonly directed at the partner, as the closest, and therefore safest recipient. Many spouses are hurt by this, in spite of understanding the reasons. Most are also suffering from the prolonged stress of caring for the patient, as well as exhaustion from taking on extra duties. The wife may have resumed work to help the financial situation, or the husband undertaken cooking and cleaning as well as his job. In addition to fatigue, the spouse is subjected to many of the changes in lifestyle suffered by the patient. Financial position may be severely affected, causing inability to meet mortgage or hire purchase commitments. Holidays may be impossible, due to poverty or medical constraints. Social life, often a joint recreation, may have to be curtailed. Contacts with both family and friends tend to decrease, due to avoidance on both sides. The family with sickness feels that it has little to offer, and the fit find contact with illness distressing and embarrassing.

4.5.2 Guilt

Guilt is usually manifested by both patient and spouse. The spouse may become lonely and isolated in a world of disablement. The resulting resentment and frustration are natural, but hard to express, because the illness is no fault of the patient. The spouse feels guilty at having complaints that are seen as trivial compared with the predicament of the sick partner. Most patients feel guilty about the effects of their illness, and regard themselves as a burden to the family, however willingly carried. This is difficult for the family to deny, since it is self-evidently true. Sadly this guilt is often expressed as anger or resentment, causing the partner to feel unappreciated. It is important for spouses or carers to maintain outside interests, partly for their own sake in order to get enough relaxation to carry on, but also to make the patient feel less guilty. It is not easy to maintain outside interests, even if good alternative care is available, or the patient able to manage alone at home. The spouse usually feels guilty in escaping from the situation, because the patient is not able to do so. The patient may also make things difficult due to some bitterness and ambivalence. It is hard to say: 'You go out and enjoy yourself', without the partner hearing '. . .and leave me here to be miserable'. Some spouses confess that while they would never let the partner down, they guiltily hope for a fatal outcome before it is too late for them to start a new life elsewhere.

4.5.3 Denial

Denial can be a most valuable coping response in chronic illness.[6] It can also lead to problems, especially when it creates a barrier between patient and spouse. If the patient is operating in an unreal world, in which he refuses to acknowledge the illness or its effects, the partner is forced to collude in the fantasy, while knowing that the true picture is very different. This prevents real communication between them. A complaint frequently heard by the social worker is that the patient is charming and uncomplaining towards hospital staff, often denying problems, yet is short-tempered and unpleasant towards the spouse. 'I wish you could see what it is like at home' is the partner's despairing comment. Many spouses attend clinic visits, just to make sure that the patient tells the doctor all symptoms. The chronically sick patient is very likely to claim that all is well, even though the spouse may know that this is not true. This seems to be due to several factors, all of which throw interesting light on the nature of chronic illness.

Firstly, as mentioned above, the patient may fear the displeasure of staff. At a later stage, when the relationship has become more equal, the patient may actually fear disappointing or hurting the feelings of staff by being less well than hoped. Many patients have commented: 'Everyone is trying so hard to help me. I do not want to let them down.'

A further fear is that complaints could lead to further admissions, investigations or another set of tablets to take. It may also be because denial has become a reflex response. If one says one is well and tries to behave as if one is well, one begins to believe it. This is a useful adaptation in everyday living, because very few people want to hear the true reply to the conventional 'How are you', least of all from someone with a severe medical problem. To fail to give a true response to the doctor, is, one would think, carrying it too far. Patients learn, however, that doctors and nurses, like anyone else, become frustrated with those who continually present complaints, especially if there is nothing that can be suggested or prescribed to cure the problem.

Finally, the concept of being well is relative, and it is easy for the patient to forget what it feels like to be fully fit. If asked 'How do you feel?', the patient will generally reply on the basis of comparison with the recent past, rather than pre-illness. A partner may notice a gradual decline in health, of which the patient is hardly aware.

4.5.4 *Effects of sexual problems*

A further source of stress may arise because the patient has neither the energy, capability nor inclination for sexual intercourse.[7] Some spouses have worried that they were no longer attractive, or that their husband or wife had found another partner. The patient may become so jealous of the spouse that every friend is seen as a sexual threat. In reality, surprisingly few spouses seek comfort elsewhere, and marriage breakdown is less common than among the general healthy population. There is an unwritten rule that one does not abandon a sick partner. Many of these marital problems could be avoided by discussion and communication, but patients are often unwilling to discuss the very topics that arouse their feelings of frustration, guilt and inadequacy.

4.6 Implications for medical and nursing staff

Respecting and encouraging patient autonomy is essential in chronic illness. There is no doubt that some doctors still feel most at ease with the unquestioning faith and compliance of the patient. More enlightened thinking is now beginning to prevail, especially in areas of chronic illness, where the essence of long-term quality of life lies in a co-operative relationship between the patient and the multidisciplinary team. Where possible, neither should be dictating terms. The patient who tries to limit the doctor's role unreasonably may arouse considerable hostility, as in the following case.

Case example: An intelligent young woman presented at the renal unit needing treatment for end stage renal failure. She told the renal physician that she wanted treatment, but no blood tests, injections, X-rays or transfusions. She also refused a transplant, which would have removed the repeated necessity for most of these procedures. This could be seen as her right to maintain control over her body and what was done to it. To the exasperated physician concerned it was like 'being asked to fly her safely across the Atlantic, but without ever looking at the control panel'. Called in to mediate, the social worker discovered that the woman had a childhood history of abuse from male relatives, leading to a fear of any invasive or painful procedure, especially if administered by a man. Some progress towards a compromise was made, through discussions with both parties, and long-term counselling initiated with the patient.

The therapeutic process is one of negotiation, balancing compliance and defiance within the bounds of safety, so that the patient can lead as full a life as possible without taking unacceptable risks. The doctor should be very aware of the patient's need to maintain a sense of control, especially when autonomy is threatened by the limitations of illness. Research suggests that the patient with an internal locus of control will tackle life with disability more effectively than one who feels at the mercy of fate, or subject to powerful others.

The patient with end stage renal failure (ESRF) needs to dialyse on a machine three times a week. Many perform this treatment at home, and therefore need to be expert in some medical techniques that would have been considered impossible for a lay person twenty-five years ago. Far from guarding and mystifying the art of medicine, it is the task of the renal physician and dialysis nurse to teach patients a complicated and potentially hazardous treatment, with the aim of creating independence. In order to live successfully as a kidney patient, one must know the rationale behind all advice. There is no place for the dictum: 'Do it because I say so. You do not need to know why'. It is not uncommon for such a patient to learn and understand more about the illness and treatment than the average general practitioner.

Risk-taking behaviour is a frequent problem for the health care team. The patient who continually jeopardises life and health by ignoring advice, or refusing help, is a source of great frustration to the good physician. Some patients use denial to the extent of making their own decision to skip several treatment sessions, not with suicidal intent, but in the belief that they can manage without. Others, especially young adults, may act out frustrations by massive dietary indiscretions, or alcoholic binges. These can be life-threatening to the renal patient. The behaviour is not directly self destructive, but often represents an attitude of ambivalence. The risk is known, but taking the risk offers a kind of excitement and discharge of tension. Those who play this Russian roulette do not wish to kill themselves, but do not value their lives very highly. It is undeniably the patient's right to make his own decisions, but medical staff find it hard to remain sympathetic in the face of risk-taking. Many referrals to the social worker are concerned with such behaviour.

4.7 The importance of multidisciplinary work in chronic illness

The most common chronic conditions, such as asthma, chronic obstructive airways disease, epilepsy, arthritis and diabetes are variably disabling from the physical point of view, but even more variably *perceived* as disabling by the patient, whose subjective experience may bear little relation to the objective severity of the illness. This is true even in more obviously disabling conditions, such as neurological disorders leading to paralysis, or renal failure needing treatment on a kidney machine. All chronic illnesses may involve prolonged contact with medical professionals, to monitor symptoms and treatment, and all may affect the family to a greater or lesser degree. The common factor is that chronic conditions will involve some long-term change or effect on the lifestyle of the patient, whether this be minor or all-embracing.

It is self evident that the needs of the whole person, rather than a medically based approach, must be considered if one is to achieve life quality in chronic illness. There is a close interaction between the illness, the disabilities and handicaps it causes, and the psychological response to these factors, which together determine the level of adjustment and rehabilitation of the patient. Financial disadvantage exacerbates all the problems of illness, and needs to be reduced as far as possible through advice on available benefits, and active advocacy. Close co-operation between medical and nursing staff, occupational and physiotherapists, dietitian, and social worker, offers the best integrated service to the patient and family.

By considering the impact of a given physical disability on each area of life, the social worker can assess likely problems that need to be addressed, and liaise with the most appropriate member of the team. There is considerable overlap within the team, partly because each member has to know the scope and role of the other members. All should also have basic understanding of the condition being treated, in order to make sound judgements. The following case example demonstrates a multidisciplinary approach.

Case example: The social worker was asked by the physician to visit the wife of a patient, who seemed to be under a lot of strain. She told the social worker that, among many problems, the worst was inability to sleep. She felt that she would be able to cope with everything if she were not so tired. The reason for her disturbed sleep was the patient's restlessness. The patient then explained that *he* could not sleep because of persistent itching. This is a common problem with renal patients due to excess levels of phosphates in the blood, normally counteracted by taking phosphate-binding tablets before meals. On enquiry, the patient admitted that he was not taking the tablets, because they were large and painful to swallow. The social worker discussed this with the physician who arranged for the patient to receive a liquid form of the medication. The dietitian was then contacted by the social worker, to check whether the patient's wife was unwittingly serving him too many high-phosphate foods. At the next team meeting it was also decided that the couple needed a holiday, which was arranged with help from the Patient's Association.

In this case, the problem presented as psychological stress in the spouse, but was traced to a medical problem in the patient. Teamwork was able largely to resolve the difficulty. The field of chronic illness benefits from a non-territorial team approach, in which the patient, as well as all the professionals involved, collaborate to the maximum and share responsibility. Some disabilities seem to present problems that are chiefly practical, and others may appear largely psychological, but the interaction between the two is so great and so complex that no useful demarcation is possible. Any practical or medical problem which cannot be satisfactorily solved may lead to anxiety and frustration or resignation and depression. Any psychological problem involving loss of confidence or low self-esteem, may affect the subject's ability to cope with life at a practical level.

The social worker's role within the team is to liaise, coordinate and communicate. At times it is necessary to act as the patient's or family's advocate, especially if patient or family feel inhibited in communicating with medical staff, or if stresses at home, work, or in relationships, have led to an uncooperative or antagonistic attitude towards staff. The social worker is more likely than other team members to know what is happening outside the hospital setting. A further role is that of lay adviser within the team. In a highly technological setting, with artificial life support systems available, doctors and nurses are well aware of the pitfalls both of over-zealous treatment to preserve life regardless of quality, and of making a decision to withdraw or withhold treatment. The social worker alone in the team, (unless a chaplain is involved), has no professional medical expertise, and is not employed by the health authority. It is therefore possible to view the situation from the standpoint of a reasonable and informed member of the general public. In this capacity, he or she can act as a sounding board for the rest of the team, who may be so closely meshed in the medical aspects that the ordinary response to the problem is temporarily obscured.

4.8 Quality of life issues and ethical dilemmas

Quality of life is a subjective concept, which can only be judged by the individual concerned. In this respect it differs from rehabilitation, which can be objectively measured on criteria such as return to work, independence of others for personal care or ability to walk a certain distance. There are those who say they are happy and contented with a life so restricted by disability that many would consider the situation intolerable. Equally there are patients with apparently minor disabilities who decide that life is not worth living. The social worker may find frustrations in helping the latter type of patient, who can find a new reason for dissatisfaction as fast as each problem is alleviated. It is possible that the patient is unaware of the real source of frustration, and needs long-term counselling. Others present problems as insoluble, when they can be overcome with practical measures such as environmental manipulation, or improvement of the financial situation through imaginative and persevering use of the benefit system. Attainable solutions should not be overlooked due to identification with the patient's hopelessness.

There will still be some patients who, in spite of all efforts, decide that life with chronic illness is not worth the struggle. This arouses strong feelings, particularly in doctors, whose training has tended to suggest that death is the ultimate failure. In conditions involving life support, such as renal failure, no active steps need to be taken. If the patient chooses to refuse treatment, and is deemed to be of sound mind, there is no real ethical dilemma. Family and medical team however, feel that they have failed the patient. The ethical dilemma occurs if the doctor overrides the patient's wishes. Treatment is then a technical assault. If spouse and family are keen to start or carry on with treatment, such 'assaults' are quite commonly undertaken, with the rationale that erring on the side of life is justifiable.

A greater dilemma occurs when a very sick patient, with a short and miserable prognosis, is not capable of informed decision-making. Medical staff are often tempted to leave decisions about withdrawal of treatment to relatives. While relatives' feelings should always be considered and respected, it is unfair to give them the responsibility for deciding the death of the patient.[8] Overwhelming guilt can then be added to bereavement. Spouses have said 'I still worry whether I really made the decision for his sake or for mine. Perhaps I was not brave enough to watch the suffering'. To avoid situations of this sort, the doctor frequently asks the social worker to discuss the matter with the family. No decisions are requested, but the social worker is able to form an opinion of the feelings and wishes of relatives, and to relay these to the doctor. If the family feel that treatment is just prolonging suffering, the doctor is then able to say that it is the medical opinion that treatment should stop. The family usually respond with relief. If the family are desperate that treatment should be continued, the doctor can suggest that this should happen for a while, and be reviewed shortly. This gives the family time to come to terms with the situation.

Patients with chronic illness present the social worker with a long-term challenge, which can be both demanding and rewarding. Not all social workers find long-term work, especially with patients who cannot become well, a satisfying task. Even modest goals may be elusive in some cases, due to unpredictable setbacks in the illness occurring when practical or psychological progress seemed attainable, or unexpected readmissions to hospital that throw months of planning into disarray. These uncertainties in medical outcome are, however, the essence of the problem faced by the patient and family, and must therefore become the province of the social worker. In order to help effectively in these circumstances, one must neither be overwhelmed by the frustrations and feelings of helplessness experienced by patients, nor expect to be able to offer answers. There are ways of mitigating the effects of illness, but there are often no tidy solutions. The patient and family benefit from the worker who can remain involved and continue to provide support, even if this is, at times, no more than acting as a safe outlet for the expression of negative feelings. Many friends and acquaintances of those facing insoluble problems withdraw both physically and emotionally as a self-protective measure. Resilience in the worker is therefore essential.

Professional detachment can be particularly hard in this area, and is not always possible, or even desirable. This applies to all disciplines working with the patient and family over the years, adding to the stress of the entire team. It is noticeable that most units dealing with chronic illness have a high turnover of staff, especially at a junior level. Those who stay, however, tend to stay for many years, due to the satisfaction of working with a close team, including courageous patients and families.

Notes

1. Millard, O. W. 'Social Aspects of Chronic Disability', in: *Continuing Care: The management of chronic disease*, J. Hasler and T. Schofield (eds), Oxford: OUP, 1984.
2. Goffman, E. *Stigma: Notes on the management of spoiled identity*, London: Penguin, 1968.
3. Townsend, P. *Poverty in the United Kingdom*, London: Allen Lane, 1979.
4. Central Council for Education and Training in Social Work, 'People with handicaps need better trained workers;, Paper No. 5, London: CCETSW, 1974.
5. Auer, J., 'Social and psychological issues of ESRF' in: *Renal Failure – Who cares?*, F. Parsons and C. Ogg (eds), Lancaster: MTP Press, 1983.
6. Johnston, M., 'Psychological aspects of chronic disease' in: *Continuing Care: The management of chronic disease*, J. Hasler and T. Schofield (eds), Oxford: OUP, 1984.
7. Stout, J. P., Auer, J., Kincey, J., Gokal, R., and Hillier, V. F., 'Sexual and marital relationships and dialysis: The patient's viewpoint', *Perit. Dial. Bulletin*, **7**, 1987, pp. 97–9.
8. Auer, J., 'Psychological aspects of elderly renal patients' in: E. Stevens and P. Monkhouse (eds), *Aspects of Renal Care I*, Eastbourne: Bailliere Tindall, 1986, pp. 200–8.

Suggestions for further reading

Anderson, R. and Bury, M. (eds), *Living with Chronic Illness: The experience of patients and their families*, London: Unwin Hyman, 1988.

Clapham, M. (ed.), *A Selection of Psycho-Social Papers*, published by BASW on behalf of the European Dialysis and Transplant Nurses Association, 1983.

CHAPTER 5

Surviving illness and loss

BRENDA BIAMONTI

Many of us suffer illness, bodily malfunction or physical trauma, are admitted to hospital and recover with little or no lasting after effects to our health or well-being. The experience, though, remains imprinted on the memory long after the body has recovered. As well as being a personal experience it can be recognised as a common human experience. This knowledge can give some insight into the profound psychological and emotional importance of such incidents. Hospitalisation, treatment and recovery are significant life events even for those people for whom the experience of being 'the patient' was only transitory. The child admitted to casualty 'to be on the safe side' following a bang on the head, or to have a minor childhood injury attended to will remember and talk about her hospital adventures long after the accident itself fades into insignificance. And who can forget the feeling of utter dependency when admitted to hospital with acute appendicitis or a heart attack? These experiences will be reminders of the vulnerability of the human body.

For people whose illnesses are not so fleeting and who suffer permanent damage or chronic ill health, the intensity of feelings must be magnified a hundredfold. Among the most poignant of these are the people who lose a visible part of their body: an eye, part of a face, a breast or a limb, and further, they may be offered a replacement part (a prosthesis). Consider the implications of this set of circumstances. To be seriously, perhaps life-threateningly ill, to lose part of one's body and to be able to see clearly that the part has gone, and then to be offered a lifeless substitute. In this chapter we will look at one particular group of people, the people who lose limbs and become 'amputees',

73

and at how they can and do survive this devastation to body and spirit.

5.1   Disablement services centres

The disablement services centres (DSC) are regional out-patient centres where individuals are assessed and fitted for prostheses (artificial limbs). Here, the new amputee can also be taught how to walk and be generally advised and helped to adapt to her changed condition. Once an amputee becomes a prosthesis wearer the centre becomes a permanent and crucial part of her life. It is here that repairs and servicing of the prosthesis will be undertaken and where any medical and physical problems associated with wearing a prosthesis will be initially assessed. In this setting the social worker can have the unparalleled luxury of being able to be present and immediately available to any patient or relative who requires her help. The social work office should be accessible and the door left open at all times during out-patient clinics except when an actual interview is taking place. A pleasant reception area with a refreshment bar can lend itself to informal meeting and talking for both patients and staff. This kind of environment encourages a relaxed atmosphere that can facilitate easier communication and complement the medical and social work interviews that would form part of the overall assessment and treatment process. It would be at such a centre that the novice would meet many others who share the same label, amputee.

5.2   Losing a limb

People lose limbs as the result of a range of unpleasant life events. A child is born with a foreshortened shinbone that ends however with a normal foot. The parents are faced with the agonising decision; should they leave the child with the discrepancy in length, which will increase as the other leg grows normally, or should they agree to the foot of the short leg being amputated so that the child can wear a prosthesis. The former choice would leave the child with an obvious deformity and pave the way for future trouble with entire body alignment, but the perfect little foot would remain. The second choice would significantly increase the opportunity, through using an artificial limb, for physical balance but would leave the child with a stump in place of a foot.

A young man rides his motor bike for an evening out with his friends. The next thing that he is aware of is the back of a bus looming into view and then, before sliding into unconsciousness, wondering how his leg came to be over there under the bus whilst he lies crumpled here, under his mangled bike. He regains consciousness in hospital glad to be alive but terrified to look under the bedclothes. He can feel both of his legs but the sensation that he is aware of in his amputated leg turns out to be the common and extremely disconcerting phenomenon of phantom feeling. Over the days he gradually emerges from a mixture of euphoria about his survival and shock at having only one leg. Will be walk again, ride his motorbike again or play football? He's alive but what will the future be like for him?

Being diabetic presents the sufferer with a range of possible symptoms, from the relatively benign to the sinister. At the more serious end of the spectrum is a condition in which sensation in the extremities of the body, typically fingers and toes, is lost or severely diminished so that minor injury is often not noticed and can easily become infected. When this occurs the wound can be very resistant to treatment, because of the poor supply of blood to the area. Take the example of a mother of a lively, sport loving family whose injured foot refuses to heal. Over an extended period of time bone too is affected and the foot becomes a painful hindrance. Amputation of the lower part of her leg becomes the only sensible treatment to remove the unsalvageable foot and to stop the pain. One can imagine some of the implications of this decision for the woman and her family.

A final example concerns the elderly person with vascular disease. This condition causes sluggish circulation that in extreme cases leads to the most unbearable pain in the lower limbs. It is a pain that affords the sufferer no relief, even with strong pain-killing drugs, during both day and night. When such an intense degree of suffering is reached the only relief lies in the amputation of the limb. When this becomes the case, the sense of gratitude that is experienced by the elderly person is matched only by their profound sense of loss.

The events that have led to the amputation are varied but

they will include a constellation of some of the following: intense pain; accompanying injuries to other parts of the body; the terrifying prospect of surgery for oneself or one's child; a period of mourning that will include the well-known symptoms of denial, bargaining, anger and so on, as described by Murray Parkes;[1] fear of the unknown and the extent of the disability; of being crippled and useless; and last but by no means least, the stigma of not having a whole body.

These things will have begun to be faced before amputation or in the very early days post-amputation, though at this stage survival will be a matter of holding on desperately to a spark of hope for the future. The social worker who works in the surgical ward of the hospital where the amputation takes place will play a crucial part in supporting and counselling through these physically and emotionally raw days. Apart from the very important practical advice about, for example financial matters, one of her main tasks will be to help the new amputee to maintain a balance between mourning the old and encouraging hope for the future. This mourning is likely to include revitalised feelings of past bereavements, for a husband or child long dead perhaps, and the intensity of these feelings can be frightening for the unprepared. The social worker will need to be able to tolerate for herself the force of some of these feelings and to guide her client calmly through them.

> *Case example*: Andrew had lost both of his parents at an early age, he had been separated from his siblings who had gone to live with relatives and he had been brought up in an orphanage. He had married and had three children but on discovering his wife's infidelity, had left them all some thirty years ago. He was now in hospital having undergone the amputation of his leg and, feeling terrified and isolated, he began to grieve this loss. He had never allowed himself to grieve when his parents had died, when he had lost his siblings or when he had left his wife and family but these old feelings rose irrepressibly to the surface and he began to mourn these earlier losses also. The social worker needed to sustain him as the floodgates opened.[2]

5.3 A changed body and a changed life

The person who suffers an amputation is not only bereaved, she is also mutilated and irreversibly changed. Initial anguish and grief are followed by a prolonged period of adjustment and of sheer hard physical work. Families and other loved ones are deeply affected by these changes and they too need their period of grieving and adjustment. This was put most succinctly by a man whose wife had recently had an amputation when he said, 'It's her leg but it's our lives'. Many a spouse loyally accompanies husband or wife on frequent and often protracted visits to the centre, involving themselves in the care and rehabilitation of their partner. Frequently it is the patient with a supportive partner or family who will recover most quickly and be able to sustain the necessary strength and persistence. Often it will be the partners in these situations who will make more use of the social worker's time than the patients themselves.

Case example: Sally, the wife of a man who had been seriously hurt in a road traffic accident, found herself taking responsibility for the financial nightmare that the accident precipitated. She was helped by the social worker to find her way through the complicated maze of state benefits and supported in her new role as unwilling head of the household. Once this relationship, based on helpfulness and trust, had been established Sally was also able to talk about some of the blame and resentment that she harboured towards her husband for not having taken adequate precautions against such financial crisis as had indeed befallen them. There was also the wife who sat quietly knitting and just wanted the occasional chat. For her the familiar presence of the social worker, who knew considerably more than her friends and neighbours about amputation, allowed her to voice her niggling doubts about the future and to seek some reassurance.

Very often it is only other amputees and professionals who will understand the problems that are very specific to being an amputee and prosthesis wearer, only they will be aware of the difficulties that can be encountered daily. This will all be a mystery to the outsider and prolonged and repeated explanations as to why this or that activity is a problem can be wearisome, boring or embarrassing for all parties. It is a great relief to be able to talk over a minor problem simply, without a long explanatory preamble. The social worker at the centre is a knowledgeable lay person who doesn't need to have the background explained. On becoming an amputee a person's path through life changes significantly, as it does when any disease or disability wreaks its particular havoc. These changes are not usually welcomed even though they might well be necessary. However people may have identified themselves in the past as parent, businessman, teacher, student, woman, man or child, for this initial period at least they are primarily identified as amputees. Until this massive change has been absorbed into the psyche and the self-image has adapted accordingly, recovery cannot be complete.

> *Case example*: Seventeen-year-old Judith had recently undergone an amputation of her leg at mid-thigh level for a bone tumour and she was coming to the end of a course of chemotherapy, as a consequence she was still somewhat fragile. She and her parents welcomed practical advice about such things as Mobility Allowance and future prospects for Judith in learning to drive a car which she was keen to do. In common with most newcomers to the centre they were still in a state of shock and needing to have the likely progress of Judith's rehabilitation repeatedly explained in increasing detail as they were able to retain yet more information. It was also absolutely plain that neither Judith nor her parents wished to talk about other implications of her illness: they were not of course pressed to do otherwise. To insist upon counselling when an invitation to do so has not been issued is to assume that the professional knows more about an individual's needs than the person does herself and indeed would be the height of arrogance.

> In situations of such vulnerability the social worker's course must always be to make clear efforts of availability and willingness to help and then, watchfully and with sensitivity to covert requests, move to the sidelines and wait. As Gerard Egan puts it:

> > They [helpers] respect their clients and express that respect by being available to them, working with them, not judging

them, trusting the constructive forces found in them, and ultimately by placing the expectation on them to do whatever is necessary to handle their problems in living more effectively .... They realise that it is a privilege to be allowed to enter the life of another person, and they respect that privilege.[3]

During the following weeks Judith was measured and fitted for her prosthesis and the social worker saw her and her parents on several occasions. From a starting point of practical help, willingly given, the work gradually moved onto more painful ground as familiarity and trust grew. At this time the main issue for Judith was in looking at and handling her stump, which she kept unnecessarily bandaged. Her antipathy towards using the term 'stump' to describe what remained of her leg bordered on the phobic. Following up the clue of the superfluous bandage it became apparent that as well as trying to cope with Judith's feelings the parents were experiencing intense guilt about their reactions. They found discussion with her on the subject excruciating difficult when they too felt similar revulsion.

The social worker was able to allow, and indeed to encourage as a normal response, what the parents had hitherto experienced as shameful and forbidden feelings. In time the intensity of these feelings subsided and were replaced by psychological tolerance, if not truly acceptance, of Judith's mutilation. In this case the daughter and parents were counselled separately. The parents feared to add to Judith's suffering by letting her know the force of their reactions to her body and she did not want to burden them further with her desperate unhappiness. The social worker, from her position of privilege, was able to offer counselling and reassurance as well as practical support to all parties.

Amputation is not a temporary affair. The precursive events may well be, as in the case of a road traffic accident, but the amputation remains a life-long fact. Amputation brings permanent change and the new amputee embarks upon a 'career' that has a language (medical and paramedical jargon) and system (the DSC) of its own. Learning the language and finding out how the system works is essential if the individual

is to become a successful amputee. Some people learn quickly
and find little to daunt them; some people deal with the system
by largely ignoring it until they need, literally, a service to their
prosthesis; and some people, particularly the frail and elderly
find it bewildering in the extreme. The social worker's role here
is one of reassurance and comfort; she will be their interpreter,
their advocate or simply, the patient's friend.[4] She will explain
repeatedly if necessary how the appointment system works, what
will happen at the next visit, when the doctor will be seen again,
and so on. All of this will have already been explained it is true,
but for the shaky old man, debilitated after several months of
hospital treatment, and confused by the unfamiliar surroundings,
it is all too much to take in.

In these situations the social worker can provide a bridge
between the institution and the person's home and social milieu.
Firstly, by being distinctly non-medical and thus providing a
sense of ordinariness, and secondly by seeking to include family
or friends in the treatment programme. This can be done by
inviting significant others into the institution so that they too
learn about the ramifications of the system and rehabilitation
programme, which in its turn will help the patient to understand
what is required. Alternatively, the social worker may make a
visit to the person's home. By choosing the latter option different
objectives can be achieved according to the circumstances. It
may for example throw some light on concerns that the elderly
person has expressed to the social worker about returning home
or indeed, confirm professional doubts. The overall message
contained within a respectful home visit should be that the
institution is interested in the person as an individual with a
social context and not simply as a passive patient.

> *Case Example*: Mr White is an example of an elderly man
> who had unfortunately been misinformed about the speed
> with which he would become mobile, and the extent to
> which he would be able to walk with a prosthesis. He
> was of the opinion that he would be given a false leg
> during the course of his first visit and, with a little practise
> would be able to put it on and walk as before. Knowing the
> length of time that he had already been undergoing painful
> treatment and the setbacks that he had encountered, the
> extent of his disappointment was heartrending to see. Mr

White's reaction was to become very angry with the social worker in her attempts to replace his misconceptions with a more accurate, though unfortunately less rosy, picture. It was crucial that Mr White was able to appreciate to some extent what his limitations with a prosthesis would be if it was to be at all useful to him. To have persisted with his highly unrealistic expectations of himself would have been to court even greater disappointment in the future. If he was to achieve any degree of mobility he would have to lower his sights. The social worker saw her job as trying to ease the disappointment that this new information brought to Mr White, maintain his hope and at the same time promote a more realistic view. Mr White was still in hospital at this point and his son and daughter-in-law, with whom he would return to live after his discharge, were invited by the social worker to accompany him to his subsequent appointments at the centre. The details of his treatment were explained in layman's terms and in this way the mystique of the system was broken for them and a truer picture of Mr White's progress and possibilities was formed. As the son and daughter-in-law began to understand more of what the future held for Mr White, they were better able to help him to understand. A very sorrowful Mr White was supported through his belated realisation that he would not be the man he was before his amputation.

5.4 *Adapting to life with an artificial limb*

The official name for an artificial limb is prosthesis. Many people have difficulty in remembering the word and indeed is it any wonder? It is a harsh word for a harsh reality. It is difficult to convey the central part that a prosthesis plays in an amputee's life. Perhaps this reflects the intense ambivalence expressed by most artificial limb users. The prosthesis itself can be seen as the very embodiment of the polarities of despair and hope that the amputee experiences. Hopeful because it enables her to walk and to regain a semblance of physical harmony; despairing because it is an ugly mechanical substitute for, and a daily reminder of, the lost part. Coming to some kind of working truce with the prosthesis involves a battle for its physical and psychological mastery, of overcoming in some way these opposing forces of dependency and distaste, of the wearer reaching a compromise within herself.

Case examples: Susan was twenty-five years old when she lost her leg.

> The first thing that I see in the morning when I wake up is THAT leaning against the wardrobe. I know that I need it if I'm going to get my little girl to school and do the shopping. I'm very grateful that I've got it and that I'm alive and have recovered; the new belt on the leg is very comfortable too, but I hate it. It reminds me that I'm not a whole woman any more.

Susan had had the misfortune to need an amputation at such a high level that she had lost in effect approximately a quarter of her body. Her recovery from the operation itself had been very painful, slow and fraught with difficulties at every stage. On sitting up for the first time for example she could not balance herself and constantly fell over to one side. When she had her first menstrual period after the amputation her body was still adapting to the onslaught it had suffered and she experienced unusual and frightening sensations. These physical problems were matched only by the psychological obstacles that she was encountering daily: to look at herself in the mirror for the first time after the amputation, to sleep with her husband again, to face friends and acquaintances who were struggling plainly with shock and embarrassment. She began the slow process of learning to walk with the prosthesis upon which she would be totally reliant for any degree of independent mobility. Prostheses feel heavy, they are literally dead weights and in use have to be lifted, or 'hitched'. Progress for Susan was drawn out and painstaking; a few minutes use a day increasing to a couple of hours after about a month when her muscles had grown used to the unaccustomed exertion. By the end of a year she had recovered from the operation and was able to wear her artificial limb for most of the day. Walking however was slow, clumsy and extremely hard work. In warm weather particularly her prosthesis, which had a stiff, padded leather corset from which the leg part itself was suspended, chafed around her middle where she inevitably became very hot and damp. The holidays in Mediterranean countries that she and her husband used to enjoy so much were now to be avoided. As is usual, fortunately in such circumstances, Susan received excellent care and advice from the nursing and physiotherapy and occupational therapy staff in the hospital. Much of the social worker's effort was directed towards Susan's mother, Edith, and her grief at the loss of her daughter's wholeness. This mother was a tower of strength to Susan and without her love and courage Susan would not have survived as well as she did. Susan's devastated husband Michael leaned heavily on Edith too; she was unshakeable in her conviction that Susan would recover and make a good life again. She gave encouragement to the two young people by the absolute steadiness and calmness of her faith and optimism. The social worker was the person to whom she could turn to rage and to ask the unanswerable, 'Why her, why my daughter?' And, as Susan struggled to walk again, the social worker shared Edith's sorrow and offered her, in her turn, hope and comfort.

Ian, aged twenty-two, was less articulate about his feelings towards his prosthesis though he began to show them clearly enough in other ways. He had lost his leg in a road traffic accident several years previously; he had made a good recovery, was very active and held down a full-time job. The social worker knew him superficially but became more involved when it was suspected that the repeated damage to his prosthesis was not accidental and it was necessary to confront him with this. It very quickly became apparent that he was deeply resentful about his dependence upon an artificial limb which he accused of always breaking and letting him down, and very angry about the loss of his own leg. Although perfectly understandable in their own right these feelings masked even deeper emotions about his parents who he felt had abandoned him at the time of the accident when he had been so damaged and vulnerable. He was usually a placid young man and his explosions, during the course of which he would literally smash his prosthesis, were terrifying to him. The social worker took on the task of helping him to recognise the different elements that were contributing to his emotional chaos, to calm his fears about being 'mental', and to encourage him towards the maturity that he had so far avoided.

With this young man we have an illustration of a common phenomenon when the prosthesis becomes the focus for all kinds of blame and hatred. In abusing his artificial limb he was not only railing against his parents and a seemingly unsympathetic world, he was also venting his feelings directly towards the very object that mocked him daily about his mutilation.

5.5   *Amputation and dying*

Much has been written in recent years, notably by workers in the hospice movement, about acknowledging death as part of life and about coping and living with it. Religious, spiritual and cultural beliefs notwithstanding, death is the end of earthly life, the life that we know, and as such causes deep and natural sorrow. Although there are exceptions of course, as a rule it is not willingly embraced, either by the dying person or those close to them.

The person who has had an amputation as a life-saving procedure will know, or at least half guess, when the attempt has not been successful; they will know that death is imminent. Death can be particularly bitter when preceded by painful and mutilating surgery, or trauma, and the social worker is often the person who will hear this painful bitterness expressed. It is felt as particularly unjust to be subjected to such aggressive treatment and still to lose one's life. As previously discussed, people will want to find a reason, a person or thing to blame and accusations of poor treatment, medical or nursing neglect or malpractice are common. This natural reaction can sometimes unfortunately make bad practice hard to pin down when it does occur and the social worker who hears such accusations walks a fine line as she supports her clients through this. She must have a sound understanding of the psychological processes at work as well as the ability to keep an open mind and an empathic heart.

The elderly person will say that it is not fair to happen at the end of a good, hard working life with no harm done to anyone; the young person will argue that the injustice is that they've not had the chance of a full life. For some people, the fact that their body will not be intact when they die assumes great importance, an expression perhaps of loss of integrity, and it is common for people to want to be buried with their amputated limb. Dreaming about the limb and searching for it are part of this longing to be intact again. This is true whether or not the individual is dying, the amputee who survives will have similar experiences. This echoes of course the 'searching' phase of bereavement as described by Murray Parkes.[5]

Family and friends will have additional difficulties of their own. The parents of a young man who had an amputation in an attempt to halt the spread of a bone cancer and who survived only a few months with no slowing of the disease, suffered the most crippling guilt. They were tormented by having persuaded him to have the amputation when he had been so terrified of the operation and of losing his leg. In some parts of their minds they believed that they were responsible for causing him unnecessary suffering and they could not forgive themselves for that. The social worker in this case could but listen and acknowledge their anguish at this stage; it was during a later stage of their grief that it became appropriate to help them to put these thoughts and feelings into perspective. This case is illustrative of the vital role that the social worker in a medical setting can play; she might well be the one person who follows through and continues to work with the bereaved after the actual patient dies.

When someone survives an accident but loses part of their body it is deeply shocking to them and their families. When this happens and the victim subsequently dies then it is devastating. A young man fell under a train that he was running to catch; both of his legs were traumatically amputated on the spot but he survived for several weeks before finally dying. His fiancée experienced not only intense grief at his death she also became prey to what is known as post traumatic shock disorder (PTSD). Although she had not been a witness to the actual event she had been intimately involved in the aftermath when her fiancé lay for several weeks in the hospital. The symptoms of this have been well documented in survivors and witnesses of large scale disasters.

PTSD can occur after a stressful or traumatic event. It involves a tendency to relive and recollect the event through dreams and flashbacks, a numbing of responses to the outside world sometime after the event, and it can cause sleep disturbance, hyperalertness, guilt, loss of memory, and an avoidance of activities that trigger memories of the disaster. If the symptoms remain untreated, they can worsen, leading to chronic depression and mental illness.

The evidence from Bradford (football stadium fire) suggests there is no correlation between the severity of the injuries and PTSD. In fact, PTSD seems to be more of a risk in the slightly injured, or those who were uninjured or only peripherally involved. Frances Clegg, a psychologist attached to the Herald Assistance Unit, believes that PTSD is not a typical psychiatric disorder. 'It is a normal reaction to the experience of highly abnormal and distressing events. Furthermore, it is not unlike reactions which are frequently developed by recently bereaved people'[6]

As is touched upon above, the symptoms are generally less well recognised when they occur in individual cases. The social worker in the medical setting will come across many such people and needs to be aware that a particular constellation of symptoms that a person describes might well constitute PTSD.

Professionals of all groups need also to be aware that if the symptoms of PTSD can be tackled at an early stage, when they are 'a normal reaction to the experience of highly abnormal and distressing events', then they need not develop into full-blown psychiatric disorders. The lesson here of course is for early and consistent intervention, a task for which no one is better placed than the hospital-based social worker when the distressing event causes hospital admission.

5.6   Life goes on

Amputation, which must seem to be one of the most devastating blows that fate can deliver, can happen, as we have seen, to anyone. Such is the resilience of human nature however that in time most people who experience amputation recover their equilibrium and continue with life as fully as they can. Once the initial trauma, which can produce unexpected effects, is over, people remain basically true to character. Personality is not a static entity and illness and disability bring changes of course, but the way in which a particular person incorporates these changes into her personality will reflect the way in which she deals with life in general. For some people, facing adversity can lead to a better understanding of themselves and of their purpose and priorities in life. The brush with mortality that an amputee may have recently experienced will remind them, as survivors, that they have much to live for and to look forward to. The losses can be counterbalanced by some gains.

> *Case example*: John was almost as badly affected by the consequences of his amputation as by the amputation itself. Although fully recovered he had grave problems in finding a job despite being only in early middle age and with solid experience. Potential employers seemed unwilling to gamble on his stamina. Equally shattering for him were the reactions of some friends who now seemed to be avoiding him. On one occasion he noticed that someone he knew quite well crossed the street as he approached. This fear of contagion is not uncommon but knowing this did not ease John's hurt. He felt, he said, like a leper. These events however were compensated for by the response of his own family.
>
> His relationships with his wife and adult daughters became closer and deeper and this was a source of great joy to him. He also made several new friends among his fellow amputees whom he met whilst attending a self help group. It was also very therapeutic for him to discover that he had a hitherto untapped capacity for supporting others.

Experiencing the near miss of severe illness leads many people to review their lives, to look for ways to make up for past mistakes, to finish unfinished business and to give themselves a second chance.

> *Case example*: Maurice had lost both legs in quick succession, paying the price of alcoholism, rough living and self-neglect. He was a tough and intelligent man when sober and he battled for almost three years with both his drinking habit, that he recognised was destroying him, and learning to walk with two artificial legs. In spite of several drinking binges when he took himself and his wheelchair off to old haunts, he returned each time to the hostel that

was his home (and refuge). After a period of drying out and hiding out he was encouraged by hostel staff, social worker and physiotherapist to attend the centre again and to work once more towards his rehabilitation. He was always faced honestly with the consequences of his lifestyle and he himself accepted this responsibility. He began gradually to review his life and to discuss with the social worker what he might do to re-make his relationships with his children whom he had not seen for about eight years, since he had begun drinking in earnest and had cut his ties with the past. Early discussions were speculative, 'What would it be like if I had kept in touch?' This was followed by, 'What would they think of me now?' and, 'I wonder what they're doing now?'. He finally made contact by letter, received a delightful reply from his daughter in America that he read and re-read. Photographs of his never seen grandchildren triggered strong, long-buried emotions and he resolved that he must stick to his abstinence if he was to regain his family and earn their longed for respect. Who knows if there will be a happy ending for Maurice but what is certain is that he worked hard at regaining some of the dignity of better times and he made ample use of his relationship with the social worker to test out his worth. One can speculate that he might not have done this had his legs not been amputated and he was literally forced to stop and think what he was doing!

The person who has laughed at life and themselves will continue to enjoy the absurdity of the human condition. There is much about the circumstances surrounding amputation that is absurd and it is an unusual person who does not see the funny side and make visual or verbal jokes at their own expense. To be able to see the comedy in the 'funny walk', to be able to laugh when an artificial limb unexpectedly detaches itself must surely be a healthy antidote when life has dealt such painful blows.

An often told story within the family concerned is about the little boy who accompanied his grandmother on her first visit to the centre. He was asked by the social worker if he had seen a false leg before and back came the contemptuous reply, 'course he had, and he'd come here to get one for his Nan, a yellow one!' Anyone who has been a patient in a hospital or who has experience of working in such a setting will know the potent therapeutic value of black humour. It enables professionals to do their work in face of what can be the grimmest of circumstances and it enables the patients to exercise some control in conditions that must sometimes seem totally out of their control.

> *Case example*: Graham had this capacity honed to a fine art. He took every opportunity to deliver outrageous remarks with a straight face and to counteract most attempts at seriousness with a well placed verbal pin prick. On one occasion, during the course of a 'serious' interview, he informed the social worker with a straight face that he was having hairs implanted on his new artificial limbs, and she was momentarily convinced! He was a farmer who had lost both of his lower legs in a farming accident and his telling of the events surrounding this sometimes took on the flavour of a farce. In this way he infused the most awful of events with the ridiculous, his familiar formula for dealing with life. Perhaps this served to diminish the nightmare quality of the accident for him and allowed him to take charge of the situation now in a way that he had been powerless to do at the time. At the same time the laughter that he engendered was cathartic for both himself and the workers who were concerned with him.

5.7   Survival and the hospital-based social worker

No chapter about surviving illness and loss can be complete without some mention of how the professional worker survives the daily onslaught of working in such a setting. It would seem, for workers who are not trained medically at all such as social workers, that an initial period of obsession with health, even hypochondria, gradually gives way to a more balanced set of feelings. The understanding that if one is to help to inculcate hope in others, one needs to be optimistic oneself, helps to sustain the worker at the saddest of times. In such a setting the social worker realises early on that 'there but for the grace of God go I'. Amputation may happen to oneself or one's partner in coming years, to one's parents tomorrow, to a son in a car accident, or a grandchild may be born with an inexplicable congenital absence of a limb. It is something that can happen to anyone and the social worker works daily with that knowledge.

The social worker will also have to confront her own memories of personal hospital experiences, of past illnesses and losses, some frightening and painful. As her clients will have to deal in some way with these resurrections, so too will the social worker. She will also become acutely aware of issues to do with authority and paternalism, the embodiments of which are the institution and the medical profession with whom she is working. The social worker in a medical setting will need to be aware of, and to resolve in some measure, any personal packages of this nature that she herself carries if she is to proceed unhindered with her work.

The daily round of working with people in the throes of shock, fear, sadness and general distress would drain or numb professional workers completely if they did not develop some safety measures for themselves. Mythology has it that doctors cut off from the feelings that 'seeing the whole person' can engender, by only seeing the component parts or the particular parts that interest them. For example, the 'chest specialist' or the 'orthopaedic surgeon'. There is truth in this as we may well have occasion to test for ourselves; it is equally true that social workers too develop mechanisms for cutting off from their clients. The capacity to project a warm, attentive manner that conceals the shutting off that is actually taking place, is something that most social workers will find that they need to call upon at times. It can be argued that some distancing is necessary to self-preservation but equally one must be aware that it is a small step from this to the emotional blunting that characterises burnout.[7] Staying emotionally receptive to painful feelings without becoming overwhelmed by them means that the social worker must be able at all times to maintain a healthy boundary between self and other, herself and the client.

The cardinal rule for this must be that social services departments recognise the particular and demanding nature of work within a hospital and provide support for their staff accordingly. The obvious call here must be for accessible and sacrosanct supervision and a stated recognition that the potential for overstress is comparable to any other branch of social work. Indeed for the young social worker it can be a source of greater stress because of the premature plunge into the realms of disease and death.

The social worker will rely a good deal on her immediate working colleagues on the ward or in the clinic who will be mostly nurses, occupational and physiotherapists and doctors. In a truly multidisciplinary working team there will be mutual support and sometimes comfort, for, despite expectations to the contrary, familiarity with the effects of suffering does not necessarily make for emotional immunity. In the best of health care settings this is now being recognised and the kinds of support outlined above encouraged. Social workers in hospitals and other health care settings should seize every opportunity to initiate such support networks where they do not already exist. Their survival may well depend upon it.

Notes

1. Murray Parkes, Colin. *Bereavement: Studies of grief in adults*. Pelican, 1988.
2. Acknowledgements to Astrid Ryan for unpublished case material.
3. Egan, Gerard, *The Skilled Helper: A systematic approach to effective helping*, Monterey, California: Brooks Cole, 1986.
4. Levenson, Ros, 'Case for the hospital-based social worker', *Social Work Today*, 15 September 1986.
5. *Op.cit.*
6. 'You bring the sadness with you', *Community Care*, 18 February 1988.
7. See, for example, Fineman, Stephan, *Social Work Stress and Intervention*, Aldershot: Gower, 1985.

Suggestions for further reading

Taylor, Rex, and Ford, Jill (eds), *Social Work and Health Care*, Jessica Kingsley, 1989.

Addison, Carole, Tolerating stress in social work practice: The example of a burns unit, *British Journal of Social Work*, **10,** 1980.

MachLachlan, Rod (ed.), 'Stress in social work', *Community Care*, no. 6, 26 March 1987.

'The team approach to the treatment of peripheral vascular disease aetiology to amputation'. Papers presented at Kings College School of Medicine and Dentistry conference 7 and 8 May 1987. (Papers available from Dulwich Medical Research Dept, tel: 01-6933 3377, ext. 3035).

CHAPTER 6

The healthy patient

MARGARET ROSS and CHRISTINE TULLOCH

6.1   Transition from healthy person to patient

Not everyone who receives medical care from a general hospital fits comfortably into our usual definitions of sick person or patient. Many people, despite being obliged to undergo the customary procedures of a hospital and to make adjustments to their social and occupational roles as a result of the medical definition of their condition, nonetheless do not suffer from any identifiable physical illness, acute or chronic and are, in the eyes of the world, 'healthy patients'.

In this chapter we shall look at two of these groups in particular – women who undergo termination of pregnancy and those who continue with a pregnancy – and at the implications for the patient, the doctor, and the social worker. As both groups of patients are female, the feminine gender will be used throughout. General statements about the role of patient would, of course, apply equally to males or females. We would wish to stress, too, that although we are here describing a very specialised area of medicine, nursing and social work, the general principles identified may be applied much more broadly.

By decision of the editors the feminine gender has been used for both social worker and doctor. In our experience, however, the patient is more likely to find that her gynaecologist or obstetrician is male rather than female.

To become a patient, the woman must first see a symptom (or set of symptoms) as a threat to her activities and relationships severe enough to make her decide to seek medical advice rather than to medicate herself or simply to accommodate herself to her symptoms (as she may well do with, for instance, back pain, varicose veins or a headache). Her decision will be influenced by a range of factors: her previous experience of medical services, for example, how frightened she is of what the doctor may say, and how important and disruptive she herself considers her symptoms and their significance to be. She may consult a doctor quickly if encouraged or pressurised by someone close emotionally to her or with some authority over her. On the other hand, she may delay seeing a doctor if she assesses her illness as one which in Goffman's words will 'stigmatise' her and thereby 'disqualify her from full social acceptance' and approval.[1] She may not relish this new, all-encompassing role as a patient which may result in the curtailment or loss of many of her normal social and occupational roles and which brings with it unwelcome feelings including anxiety, uncertainty, helplessness, dependency and regression – feelings which run counter to the principles of autonomy and self-determination which form an integral part of her adult identity.

In order to become familiar with the norms, values and expectations of her new role as a patient, the woman is obliged to undergo a process defined by sociologists as 'secondary socialisation'. If she is admitted to hospital or even if she simply receives medical attention as an out-patient, she becomes in effect a 'non-person' – what Goffman describes as a 'serviceable object who is shaped, codified and fed into the administrative machinery of the establishment to be worked on smoothly by routine operations'.[2] Ordinary behaviour – drinking, eating, urinating and defaecating, etc. – may be restricted and/or closely monitored by hospital personnel, so the patient is unable to distance and protect herself from the institution. In addition, she faces separation from her familiar surroundings and from family and friends who must also accept the institution's authority and abide by its rules if they are not to risk exclusion from it. The patient may suffer pain or discomfort, be stripped of her own 'identity equipment', as Goffman called it – make-up, clothes, jewellery, false teeth, spectacles, etc. – and be obliged to adopt abnormal dress (theatre gowns, elastic stockings, etc.). She may also have to accept into her body or on to its surface a variety of unaccustomed and often frightening and painful items of medical equipment – intravenous needles, pills, sutures, catheters, etc., administered by staff whose manner of dress defines their role and status within the hospital hierarchy.

Because of the medical definitions applied to the situation and the freedom from ordinary social conventions which results, staff are granted the right of access to certain taboo areas of the patient's body which might otherwise be interpreted as assaults upon her person. Because she cannot 'leave behind for servicing' the malfunctioning part of her body, the patient must reveal, sometimes to a succession of hospital personnel, the most intimate areas of her body and the most private details of her social statuses and behaviour, past and present. Given that she cannot use her body in the usual fashion while it is being repaired, and that as a new patient she must somehow succeed in setting aside the 'presenting culture' of her familiar world and her whole previous way of life and the usual image of herself which she presents to others, it is hardly surprising that she may feel embarrassed and disorientated.

An example is the woman undergoing a cervical smear. This procedure, although quick and usually not unduly painful, may prove for many women distasteful and humiliating. Anxiety for the patient is heightened, too, by the prospect that an abnormality may be discovered which will destroy her image of herself as a healthy woman.

The gains the patient makes which help to counterbalance the 'symbolic cost'[3] of becoming a patient include relief from the crisis which her symptoms have provoked, and the reassurance that her illness has been medically defined and thus recognised as legitimate and requiring treatment. Her status as a sick person is therefore validated so that others now know how to behave towards her and will allow her temporary exemption without penalties from at least some of her usual role responsibilities. She has acted in accordance with our lay person's assumption that it is undesirable and indeed socially deviant to be ill and that the patient, as a sick person, is obliged therefore to seek competent help and to co-operate in the process of becoming well again.

6.2   The role of the doctor

If the social worker is to work effectively and harmoniously alongside the doctor, it is imperative that she have some understanding of the way doctors are trained to view themselves, their patients, and their position in the hospital hierarchy. The doctor plays a complementary role to that of the patient, without whom she could not perform as a doctor. She must make a diagnosis of the problem, determine the most appropriate treatment, and secure the patient's agreement and co-operation. She may have to try to balance the interests of an individual patient against the good care of a large group of patients; the present versus future needs of a patient; the patient's interests versus the needs of medical research and medical students. The doctor may try to cope with these conflicts by developing a belief in her own wisdom and individualism – a belief with which the patient may well collude as it makes it easier for her then to trust the doctor to whom she has 'handed over' her body.

In order to distance herself from the embarrassing, distasteful procedures to be performed, and to minimise the risk of becoming personally involved with patients, the doctor brings to her work what Parsons terms a sense of 'affective neutrality' or objectivity. She will also try to employ the principles of 'universalism' (all patients are of the same value) and 'functional specificity' (the doctor is concerned only with those matters which are of direct medical relevance to the patient).[4]

For some doctors, the provision of medical care to a woman seeking abortion may be distasteful and difficult. It may seem that this is not 'proper medicine' and that to play a complementary role to this group of patients runs counter to the skills and values of the medical profession. However small the risk may be, the doctor is aware that by her intervention, a healthy woman will be exposed to risk – e.g. of uterine perforation or an adverse reaction to the anaesthetic. If the woman seems sure of her decision and is asking for the doctor's co-operation rather than her advice, the doctor may feel reduced to the level of a technician – a far cry from the dominant, paternalistic stance which doctors by training and societal expectation have in the past tended to adopt. To agree to a request for abortion gives the doctor only one possible course of action rather than the range of options – medication, X-rays, physiotherapy, etc. – which can be presented to most patients. (Similar clear-cut requests by other groups of healthy patients would include those for sterilisation, reversal of sterilisation, gender realignment, and treatment of primary infertility).

The doctor may face conflict between the obligation and wish to help an individual patient, and her duties as an agent of the state in the endorsement and administration of the Abortion Act 1967. The nature of this Act means that, unless a doctor takes a strictly medical interpretation of the risk to health and accepts referral only of women who are physically or mentally seriously ill or where the foetus has been diagnosed as having a handicap which is incompatible with life, she will be obliged to look at the whole patient and her life circumstances, assessing 'a complex set of psychological and social variables'.[5] The principles learned as a medical student – of universalism, affective neutrality and functional specificity – may well prove in this case not to offer a complete and reliable framework for decision-making.

The woman who continues with her pregnancy may likewise view the doctor's role very differently from the doctor herself. Despite the skills and technical expertise which the hospital doctor offers to the antenatal patient the latter may – unless she has pre-existing medical problems or a particularly difficult pregnancy – feel more comfortable in her relationship with her general practitioner and community midwife, both of whom she is likely to see more often and in the less austere surroundings of her own home or local health centre.

6.3   Women requesting a termination of pregnancy

The woman who seeks a termination of pregnancy fits Western societies' stereotypes neither of the happily expectant mother nor of the sick person who deserves medical care and the approval and support of those around her. Because her attitude to her pregnancy is seen as incongruous and undesirable, she runs the risk of losing others' acceptance of her and of being labelled as socially deviant. She will be looked upon as having the same attributes as other women who share the same stigma – an uneasy alliance if she has been a harsh judge of such women in the past.

> *Case example*: Pat R. (23), pregnant as the result of erratic contraception at a time of instability in her long-standing relationship, felt ashamed of her predicament, especially as she had previously made no secret of her contempt for women who were 'careless, and who then behaved even more badly by asking for an abortion'. To find herself in the

same situation and to feel she must make the same request highlighted for this woman the need to re-examine, with the help of the social worker, her prejudices, assumptions, and moral judgements in the context of her own life situation.

A dilemma facing the woman seeking an abortion is that she needs to see herself as sick and in need of medical help, but in this case she may well *not* identify herself as sick, or she may (often correctly) imagine that hospital personnel will not. She may consider herself responsible for her own problem and therefore not deserving of help. (This type of moral evaluation is, in fact, common in our definition of illness, e.g. lung cancer as the just deserts of the smoker, AIDS of the homosexual, an unplanned pregnancy of the woman who 'gives herself too readily' to men.) That being so, she may feel guilty at her consumption of limited, valuable resources – the doctor's time and skills, the nurse's care, a hospital bed, operating theatre time, etc. She may feel selfish when comparing her own plight with that of others (e.g. children with leukaemia, the elderly victims of assault, etc). She may see herself virtually as 'untouchable' so that she imagines her care will be distasteful to hospital personnel and will bring them no sense of pride or satisfaction in their work. The social worker's role here may be that of helping the woman explore her feelings of guilt and shame so that she may separate her fantasy of other's opinion of her from her own feelings about herself.

To enter the hospital system and to be defined as a patient, the woman seeking an abortion must normally first consult her general practitioner or a family planning doctor (perhaps choosing a specific doctor whom she feels will be gentle in her treatment of her and understanding of the reasons for her request) and secure referral to a hospital out-patient clinic (where she is likely to have no choice as to which doctor she will see nor of which gender). The set routines at clinic may be necessary for the smooth running of the system but may enhance the doctor's professional autonomy at the expense of increasing the woman's anxiety and sense of depersonalisation.

Out-patient clinics may well be held in a maternity hospital, an environment which is likely to increase the woman's feelings of shame and embarrassment, and confirm her expectation that some form of punishment for her deviance is inevitable and that

obstacles will be presented to add to her discomfort or to test her
resolution.

> *Case example*: Carole F. (28) was extremely distressed to
> discover that the gynaecology out-patient clinic she must
> attend was held in the same maternity hospital in which
> she had happily delivered her baby four years previously.
> She saw this as a deliberate policy to make the process of
> securing an abortion more difficult. As an antenatal clinic
> was held at the same time, she felt out of place, isolated,
> and the only woman who was not happy to be pregnant.
> She was sure that everyone could guess why she was there
> and waited in terror for something to be said or done which
> would identify her beyond all doubt as a woman planning
> to terminate her pregnancy. Having explored these painful
> areas with the social worker, Carole could then move on to
> a re-identification of the factors which made a termination
> of pregnancy the right decision for her at this time.

The woman may, on the other hand, look for obstacles but find
none.

> *Case example*: Tracey L. (20) had come to clinic fully
> prepared to be rebuked and humiliated and to have her
> reasons for requesting an abortion discounted as not
> good enough. She found it hard to believe that hospital
> personnel would treat women making such a request with
> compassion and consideration.

The woman may welcome and accept this approach or she
may conclude that the importance for her of this life crisis
has not been recognised, and any doubts she may have about
terminating the pregnancy have been ignored, making it almost
impossible for her to raise them herself. If she considers some
form of punishment for her deviance inevitable and necessary,
a lack of obstacles before the abortion may lead her to believe
that punishment has merely been deferred.

> *Case examples*: Diane W. (17) was referred by her GP for
> counselling six months after a termination of pregnancy.
> Diane had waited for hospital personnel to treat her unkindly,
> for pain, or for rejection by her friends. When none of
> these occurred she became increasingly uncomfortable and

tense. When she had an opportunity during counselling to list again the reasons which had led to her request for abortion and could accept their validity, and when she had examined the assumptions she had made about the way she would be treated as a patient, she was able to begin to put the crisis into perspective and to use the self-knowledge she had gained in her approach to other challenging situations.

Mandy P. (22) miscarried a wanted pregnancy at nine weeks. She saw this as a direct punishment for the abortion she had undergone two years earlier. As she had not told her husband about the abortion which had taken place before they met, her sadness was intensified by feelings of shame and regret despite the fact that she had requested the abortion only after much soul-searching and consideration of the alternatives.

The availability of a social worker at out-patient clinics ensures that distressed women are referred at this stage and are given the opportunity to express the ambivalent feelings they may have. Fantasies can be explored, concrete information secured, and ongoing social work support offered.

If abortions are carried out in a day surgery unit, the woman will find it difficult to set up her own personal space marked out by the flowers, cards and fruit which normally indicate such things as the length of her stay in hospital and the number of people by whom she is considered important. She is unlikely to find the sense of camaraderie and the sharing of hospital experiences which are an everyday feature of many other wards. (These last two are also largely absent among patients in intensive treatment units and on wards for very confused patients although in this case visitors to both groups may set up relationships amongst themselves.) In fact, the woman undergoing an abortion may be relieved that there are few personal identity symbols in the ward and that her fellow patients rarely attempt to establish personal relationships with her. At the same time, the efficient detachment with which the range of set procedures is carried out and the difficulty this detachment may give rise to for the woman who longs in silence for reassurance from staff or fellow patients, may accentuate her feeling of loneliness and her fearful unfamiliarity with the complex bureaucratic organisation of a large hospital. Again, ready access to a social worker may help the woman as she explores and expresses her mixed feelings about the process she is undergoing.

Each method of abortion may, by its nature, cause the woman anxiety and distress, however irrational and unwarranted her reaction may seem to hospital personnel, given their greater familiarity with, and understanding of, the procedures performed. For some women, the idea of general anaesthesia arouses fears that they will not be completely unconscious but will be unable to alert theatre staff to their plight, or at the other extreme that they will never regain consciousness. They may harbour anxieties about what they may say or do whilst not in full control of all their faculties. An abortion under local anaesthesia may bring fears about pain, distasteful sights, and the same of finding oneself unable to tolerate the procedure once it has begun. The use of prostaglandins in mid-trimester abortions also evokes fears of pain – in this case over a prolonged period – and one's ability to cope emotionally with a distressing procedure which bears ironic similarity to labour but which lacks its final reward and sense of fulfilment.

The woman undergoing termination of a pregnancy where foetal abnormality has been diagnosed faces the possibility of a particularly distressing experience. However gently and considerately she is treated by hospital personnel, nothing can lessen the immediate shocked impact of discovering that a serious foetal abnormality has been discovered and that abortion is advised on medical grounds. The pregnancy may be greatly wanted and far advanced. There may be little time for the woman (and her partner) to adjust to the devastating news before the abortion must be carried out. The woman may face the additional agony of having to make a decision about abortion where her medical advisers cannot identify with absolute certainty the precise gravity of the handicap. She may feel guilty that *she* is healthy whereas her foetus is not, and in an attempt to establish a cause of the abnormality she may examine critically her diet, recent activities, and so on, blaming herself for supposed thoughtlessness or self-indulgence. She may see herself as incapable of producing a healthy baby in the future.

Case example: Peta B. (39) was pregnant for the first time. The foetus was diagnosed at eighteen weeks as suffering from severe chromosomal abnormalities and an abortion was performed. Peta talked sadly of her decision that this should be her only pregnancy as she felt she could not cope emotionally with the risk in any further pregnancies of abnormality due to her age or other factors.

The possibility of securing a mid-trimester abortion is essential for women like Peta, where foetal abnormality cannot be diagnosed with certainty any earlier. Its availability is vital too for other women – those who because of extreme youth and/or fear of the social consequences have refused to admit even to themselves the reality of a pregnancy until an advanced stage, or those who because of irregular menstrual cycles, perhaps as they approach the menopause, have genuinely not realised they were pregnant for some considerable time.

If the upper time limit for performing abortions is reduced, it may be expected that NHS hospitals and private clinics will, as at present, leave a margin between their own upper limit and that established by law. Many women currently able to have a mid-trimester abortion will, therefore, be obliged to continue with their pregnancies.

It seems inevitable that increased resources, both statutory and informal, will then be required. Some women may choose to have their babies adopted, thus making necessary the diversion of more social work time for the selection and preparation of potential adopters as well as for the counselling and support of the biological mother both during and after the pregnancy. For the woman – often little more than a child herself – who decides to keep her baby, the combined resources of the education department, social services, Social Security, and the Health Service may be required if she is to be able to provide a safe, adequate environment for her baby. The birth of increased numbers of handicapped babies as a result of the lowering of the upper time limit for carrying out abortions will similarly require long-term, expensive input from at least some of the statutory services if the concept currently so much in vogue of community care is not to become a euphemism for unsupported care by exhausted, beleaguered families.

The fact that she has undergone a termination of pregnancy remains for the woman a permanent aspect of her personal biography, and one which requires of her that she adjust emotionally to the 'spoiled identity' which this stigma has caused, construct a new image of herself, and form a new view of her world. At the time of the abortion she may find that others, disapproving of her, may either continue to make heavy demands on her which she may find intolerable, or may not return to her after the abortion the social roles she has been unable to perform during the crisis. If she has chosen instead not to disclose information about the abortion to others, her temporary role as a patient which prevents her from performing her usual social roles will go unrecognised and she may be considered untrustworthy and 'AWOL'. She must live too with the risk that her secret will be unexpectedly revealed against her wishes, for example if she later meets a woman who was a fellow patient, and the knowledge that she cannot erase the written medical record of the event.

Happily for many women the experience of abortion, although almost inevitably accompanied by feelings of sadness, does not produce long-term emotional or relationship problems. Where the woman has been respectfully treated by hospital personnel, given adequate counselling and assured of adequate continuing support, and where the disruption to her roles is kept to a minimum, she may emerge from this crisis with an enhanced confidence in her ability to surmount challenges and the reassurance that she is still valued, respected and loved by those whose opinion is important to her. The attitude of the doctor and the social worker may well be crucial in helping to secure this happy resolution.

6.4   The pregnant woman

6.4.1   The changing face of maternity services

The care of the pregnant woman has changed dramatically during the course of this century. Eighty years ago, there was little antenatal care and the majority of women gave birth at home in conditions which were far from satisfactory. Today, women are monitored throughout their pregnancies and most babies are born in hospital with all the assistance of modern technology. In one English county, for example, in 1988 only 48 babies were born at home compared with 6,370 delivered in hospital. The effects of this change can be clearly seen in the fall of the infant mortality rate from 150 per 1,000 live births in 1900 to the rate of 8.9 per 1,000 in 1988. This change is also mirrored in the fact that as late as 1932, there was one maternal death for every 238 live births (Registrar General Statistical Review for 1932) in contrast to 1980 when only 68 maternal deaths were registered, a rate of 0.11 per 1,000 births. The decline in the maternal mortality rates resulted from several factors – the discovery of the sulphonamide drugs for the treatment of puerperal sepsis, later followed by the discovery of penicillin and increasing use of blood transfusions for women who haemorrhaged. There has also been a general improvement in social conditions – better housing, less poverty and unemployment – which have all contributed to greatly improved health among women of child-bearing age. All these factors have played an important part in the vast improvements which have taken place in the maternity services during the past eighty years. Childbirth is now considered to be a normal function which carries little risk for the average healthy woman.

There are, however, those who feel that the increasing emphasis upon the hospital as the only place for babies to be born safely may detract from the woman's experience of childbirth. In her book *The Captured Womb*, Ann Oakley states that 'hospitals, by aligning normal parturition with the confinement of the sick, created a medical label for pregnancy'.[6] This has meant that women who regard pregnancy as a perfectly normal condition, have increasingly become subject to closer medical surveillance and intervention both in the antenatal period and during labour. The healthy patient is made to feel that her condition is in some way pathological and this is paralleled by the conflict between doctors and midwives over the care of the pregnant woman. In her introduction to *The Midwife Challenge*, Sheila Kitzinger defines the role of the midwife as being 'able to diagnose deviations from the normal, to intervene and to refer to the obstetrician when necessary, but her important skills are in maintaining and supporting the normal physiological processes of birth'.[7] Midwives have had a long struggle to maintain their professional status and have increasingly seen themselves in conflict with the medical profession in their efforts to be seen as the 'experts' in normal childbirth. The Association of Radical Midwives in a paper *The Vision* defines the objective of the maternity services as 'a safe, sensitive service that sees childbirth as a part of life, not as a disease'[8] There has also been an increasing impact upon the provision of obstetric care by the consumers themselves. The National Childbirth Trust and the Association for Improvements in the Maternity Services (AIMS, founded in 1960) have fought hard to ensure 'the right of the mother to experience normal physiological childbirth without interference unless she wants it or there are clear indications that it is needed'.

Although there has been a trend for the majority of women to give birth in hospital, there has also been an increasing tendency for the amount of time spent in hospital following normal delivery to become ever shorter. The average stay for postnatal women in some maternity hospitals is now only 3.8 days. New patterns of care have emerged because of the cuts in the NHS budget. Although there will always be a hard core of patients who do need long-term antenatal admission because of underlying medical conditions or complications with the pregnancy itself, there is a growing awareness that a patient's social circumstances, particularly if she has other young children at home, make life very stressful if she has to be admitted. It has been shown that a number of these women can be dealt with using a system of daily assessment at the hospital which avoids the need for admission.

The role of the social worker within the obstetric field must, in essence, differ from that of her colleagues working in other hospital settings. Pregnancy is, by definition, a self-limiting condition and the majority of women who are expecting a baby do not regard themselves as ill. It is, however, for many women a major turning point in their lives which will involve changes in their relationships and social circumstances. This is especially so for the woman who finds herself with an unplanned pregnancy. She may have decided, following counselling, not to seek termination but it is a decision which can have profound consequences. The birth of a baby can be a crisis for some, especially if the baby is born prematurely or is handicapped or stillborn. Although the mother may be seen as the patient, she and her new baby are part of a family and this may have implications not only for her own parents but also for the father and his family. The age of the mother can range from a young teenager to a woman in her middle 40s and for each the problems will be different. Within this context, the role of the social worker can range through a spectrum from helping someone to resolve complex feelings about whether she should place her child for adoption to supporting a mother through the birth and death of a handicapped child and yet also dealing with the more mundane problems of housing and welfare benefits.

One of the most important tasks for the maternity social worker is the screening and monitoring of mothers who are likely to be a cause for concern once their babies have been born. Ounsted and colleagues, in a paper entitled 'The fourth goal of perinatal medicine' put forward the theory that it was possible to predict at a very early stage following delivery that if a mother appeared to be having significant problems in bonding with her baby, then there was an increased risk of subsequent problems and even child abuse.[9] Many of these mothers are likely to be young, single and unsupported. During the past decade, there has been a rise in the number of babies born to single women to about one quarter of the total. It is, however, important to recognise that the increase has been due mainly to births outside marriage but to couples who are cohabiting in a stable relationship rather than in those which are registered by the mother on her own. In 1986, 284 girls (5.4 per cent of the total) under the age of 20 gave birth in one major maternity hospital. The majority of girls in this category are single and still live at home.

For most of them, this is the best solution especially if they have a good relationship with their parents. There is help at hand to look after the baby and support from the extended family. There are, however, a minority of young mothers who are already living away from home in places where children are unwelcome or whose relationships with their families have broken down, sometimes as the result of divorce and the remarriage of one or both parents. If they become homeless the local authority, under the provisions of the Homeless Persons' Act 1977, has a duty to rehouse them, but in practice this usually means that they are put into cheap hotels with no cooking facilities. It is this group who are particularly vulnerable and may need considerable social work support.

Case examples: Heather had lived with her father and stepmother since her parents had divorced eight years earlier. There were already tensions within the household prior to the birth of Heather's baby but the situation broke down completely after she went home and she became homeless. She was placed in bed and breakfast accommodation by the housing department and was referred to a community social worker because of concern about her ability to care for her baby adequately. Arrangements were made for her to attend a family centre on a regular basis to improve her mothering skills and she was introduced to a group of other young single mothers to help lessen her feelings of isolation. She was also able to re-establish some contact with her family with the help of her social worker.

Another girl whose situation was even more complicated was Sharon who was 18. She had already had one termination of pregnancy and then subsequently became pregnant again. Her mother had died the year previously and Sharon was still grieving for her. Her relationship with her father had broken down and in the year before she became pregnant, she had moved from one bedsit to another. She was also unemployed and living on Income Support. She was finally admitted to hospital because of concern about the growth of the baby and at this stage was homeless. During her time in hospital she needed to talk at length about her mother's death, her social isolation and her attitude towards the new baby whom she saw, primarily, as satisfying her need for something of her own to love. Her housing problems were resolved when she was allocated a room in a hostel for single girls and their babies. She was referred to an area team social worker on discharge because of her need for continuing support and to link her into the resources in her area. Sharon in many ways typifies the isolated, emotionally deprived adolescent who either becomes pregnant or who decides to continue with an unplanned pregnancy because she sees this as a solution to her problems.

One of the difficulties for the social worker in a large regional unit is the problem of following up her client. The need to ensure continuity of care will bring her more closely in touch with social workers in the area teams than many of her hospital colleagues. Liaison with social work teams in the catchment area of the hospital is also vitally important where there are worries about whether a baby is likely to be at risk. Very often, girls about whom there is concern are already known to a social services department and previous children may have been received into care. If the decision is taken, following a case conference, to apply for a new-born baby to be made a ward of court or to apply for a place of safety order on its behalf, midwives and doctors can find this hard to accept since all their training and expertise is dedicated to the care of mother and child. It can be very difficult for them to behave normally with a mother when they are aware that it is unlikely that she will be allowed to keep her new-born infant. The intrusion of the social worker as an authority figure into this setting often requires considerable liaison with staff in order to handle the situation in the most sensitive way possible.

Case example: Carol, (19) had been brought up in care since the suicide of her mother when she was 7. She had had a variety of foster placements which had broken down and as soon as she was old enough to leave care, she had led an extremely unsettled existence, moving from place to place and living in a variety of temporary accommodation. She had already had one child and although she had been given maximum support in a mother and baby home, she had neglected the child who was eventually taken into care. Carol, who was also drinking heavily, was aware of the concern of social services before she delivered and had been told of their plans to make the baby a ward of court. In the event, the baby was born prematurely and was admitted to the special care baby unit. Carol promptly took her own discharge. She did not come back even to see the baby. In a situation such as this, the hospital becomes the backdrop for the resolution of a social crisis simply because this is where the mother receives her medical care.

6.4.2   *The crisis of concealed pregnancy*

In his book, *Person-in-distress: On the bio-social dynamics of adaptation*, Hansell defines a crisis as 'any rapid change or type of encounter which is very much outside a person's usual range of experience'.[10] This definition is particularly applicable to the woman who presents with a concealed pregnancy. There is no universally accepted definition of this condition, but in general terms it is applied to a mother who has not booked or received any antenatal care before twenty-eight weeks. It also includes a small group who proceed to full term without discovery and one or two who take the situation to the ultimate extreme and deliver themselves. This is indeed a crisis and one which can be traumatic for the families involved as far-reaching decisions have to be made about the future of the baby. In a study of about forty girls made by the author and as yet unpublished, two distinct groups appeared to emerge.

The first group consisted of girls who had known for some time that they were pregnant but who for various reasons – fear, embarrassment, ignorance or apathy had not sought antenatal care. One young Irish girl, Carmel, arrived at her doctor's surgery in a state of advanced labour and was delivered by her astonished GP. She had been aware of her pregnancy and although she had made no preparations for the baby, her family rallied round and she took to motherhood like a duck to water. Another girl, Tracey, however, arrived unannounced in the labour ward and following delivery told the staff that she wanted to have the child adopted. He was her second baby and as a single, unsupported mother she felt unable to cope with him. She had been too ashamed to admit to her family and friends that she wanted to give him away and had succeeded in hiding the fact of her pregnancy.

The second group of mothers who conceal their condition seem to be genuinely astonished when they discover that they are far advanced in pregnancy, and although it is hard for the average person to understand, they appear to be able to deny the physical changes completely. This group seem to find it much more difficult to bond with their babies and it would seem that antenatal acceptance is a necessary part of this process. One young nurse, Anne, came into hospital in labour and was initially in a state of shock following delivery. She needed considerable time spent in counselling before she could accept the reality of the baby and make plans for his eventual adoption. In a situation such as this, it is important for the social worker to be readily available and able to devote enough time to the crisis.

It is also important to see the girl in the context of her family. The majority of girls who conceal their pregnancies are in the age group 15–21 and their own mothers frequently find it difficult to come to terms with their new status as grandmothers. They may have feelings of anger towards their daughters but also feelings of guilt that they have failed to protect them adequately. One is often told, 'I did not think my daughter's relationship with her boyfriend had gone that far'. They may also feel that they should have been aware, like the mother who had been unable to understand why her daughter had refused to remove her large, baggy T-shirt during a family holiday in Spain. The girl may still be seen as a child by her family and fathers, in particular, may find it difficult to accept that their daughters are sexually active. The arrival of the new baby can cause a distortion in family relationships especially if the grandmother takes over the role of mother. One still occasionally comes across cases where a child has not been aware that the person it has always regarded as a sister is, in fact, its mother. Considerable time may need to be given in counselling all the members of a family in a situation such as this.

6.4.3   The sick patient

Although, as has already been discussed, the majority of women do have normal pregnancies and deliveries, there are some conditions which may mean that the woman will need hospital admission for some time prior to the birth. A woman with placenta praevia (low-lying placenta) may have to come in because she is at risk of haemorrhage which could put not only the baby's life but also her own in danger. A mother who is a diabetic or has some other pre-existing disease may also need close monitoring which can result in the need for admission. This kind of situation can impose great stress upon the whole family, because not only is there concern about the mother and baby but there may also be problems about the care of other young children. There may be a threat that the husband will lose his job with resulting financial crisis if there is no member of the extended family who can help.

The fact that specialised monitoring resources such as ultrasound are now mainly centred in major hospitals, means that the most appropriate place for a patient to be may be at some distance from her own home. The hospital social worker may need to mobilise resources in the community in order to help. It may be that arranging for child-minding or even fostering will be needed and financial assistance can enable a family to visit most frequently. The patient herself may also find it difficult to cope with long periods as an in-patient. She may feel a variety of emotions – guilt because she cannot look after her other children, anger towards the unborn child because of the problems which are being caused and frustration at what she may feel is imprisonment by the hospital. She may find it difficult to express these feelings to medical and nursing staff in case she seems ungrateful for the care they are giving her to ensure a safe outcome to the pregnancy. The social worker because she is not directly involved can act as listener and support and act as liaison if necessary.

There is also another darker side to work in a maternity hospital, for not every mother does give birth to a normal, healthy baby. Some babies are premature and need admission to the special care baby unit, some are handicapped and a few even die.

Case example: Rachel's baby was born with severe spina bifida and hydrocephalus. Although she was aware of this, as the baby's condition had been diagnosed by scan during her pregnancy, she was still hoping against hope that he would survive. The baby lived for only three days but she was able to spend this time with him, look after him and finally be there when he died. The social worker was the only member of the hospital team who had been there consistently throughout all the different stages and because of this, she was able to help her express her feelings of grief at the loss of this much wanted baby. It can be very difficult for a mother who regards herself as a normal healthy person to accept that she has given birth to a child who is sick or damaged. This subject will be further discussed in a later chapter.

6.5   The role of the social worker

By training, outlook and experience the social worker has a valuable role to perform in work with pregnant women, and particularly with those who express ambivalence about their pregnancies. The social worker offers non-judgemental, non-directive counselling which in the case of the woman requesting a termination of pregnancy is not tied up in the legalities of the abortion decision but complements the work done by the rest of the health care team. She is trained to help the distressed, uncertain woman to explore her feelings and is able to tolerate the expression of powerful, negative feelings (e.g. anger and fear) without trying to minimise or invalidate them. In this safe environment, the pregnant woman may feel able to share information which is very relevant to her current dilemma but previously hidden from medical personnel.

> *Case examples*: Angela B. (17), was happy at the safe arrival of her baby but her pleasure was marred by the mutual animosity between her mother and boyfriend, both of whom wanted to name the baby and to make major decisions about his care. Angela was uncomfortably aware of her own role as mediator and 'casting vote' between this warring couple. With the help of the social worker, Angela was able to talk honestly with her mother and boyfriend about the unhappiness and anxiety she was experiencing, and her resolution that she herself would make the final decisions about the baby's care and upbringing. The two recognised that they had ignored Angela's feelings in their determination to outmaster each other, and promised to try to resolve any future disagreements by discussion and compromise. As Angela and her boyfriend were living with Angela's mother, however, it would be unrealistic to assume that the relationship problems would from then on be easily and completely resolved or that there would be no further role for the social worker.
>
> June F. (18) had a mother who was exerting pressure on her to terminate her pregnancy whereas she herself wished to have the baby. Only when she was admitted for the abortion and, noted by nursing staff to be withdrawn, was referred to the social worker for counselling, did the true situation emerge.

Hilary R. (19) confided to the social worker soon after her abortion that she had been made pregnant by her uncle, her abuser for eleven years. Although she had never before revealed this secret to anyone, the crisis provoked by her pregnancy and admission to hospital made it impossible for her to maintain any longer the pretence of being a normal young woman with good family relationships. With professional help, the long and painful process towards recovery from the abuse could then begin.

The social worker's knowledge of the options available to a pregnant woman who is considering abortion and her familiarity with Social Security benefits, adoption procedures, possibilities for securing accommodation, and so on, should ensure that the woman is well furnished with the information she requires to make a considered decision about her pregnancy. The social worker's client-centred approach encourages her to look with the woman at her problems and their possible solutions as these appear to her in the context of her roles and relationships, her values and her aspirations. Counselling offered can be flexible in terms of its duration and the number of people whom the woman chooses to bring with her. Where the woman decides to continue with her pregnancy, this valuable early link can then continue and develop so that emerging or ongoing problems can be tackled before they reach crisis proportions.

In work with pregnant women, as in work with other patient groups, the social worker's perspective and that of the doctor may at times clash, requiring compromise by both and a willingness to re-examine old assumptions and prejudices. The social worker may face additional conflict between loyalty to the primary health care team as a whole and loyalty to her employing authority. Working as she does in a secondary setting, the social worker is, however, well placed to recognise the problems the patient may encounter in this alien setting – the jargon and frightening procedures, one's fantasies and illogical fears as a patient, the difficulties of reconciling the needs of other family members with the demands made of the patient by the hospital system, etc.

The social worker can therefore act as a mediator and interpreter between patient and hospital personnel, relaying the woman's feelings and fears to the rest of the team and ensuring that information and reassurance (which in her anxiety the woman often does not hear on first telling) are repeated by the appropriate member of the team.

Couples attending fertility clinics may very appropriately be defined in most instances as healthy adults who for some reason, known or unknown, are having difficulty in conceiving or in carrying a pregnancy to term. The social worker, as a member of the hospital team but not directly involved in the administering of treatment, is uniquely placed to offer help to these couples. The stress imposed on their relationship by what may prove to be years of investigations and treatment may be intolerable. Some procedures may raise ethical issues which a couple need to explore in counselling. Ultimately, some couples will welcome the skilled help of a social worker as they decide to discontinue treatment and to redefine themselves as a couple who have not had (and who will never have) a baby born of their relationship.

The social worker can offer a specialist service to community-based agencies – general practitioners, schools, etc. – who can then refer the woman requesting abortion counselling or experiencing socio-medical problems during a continuing pregnancy to a named person preferably even before her entry into the main hospital system at out-patient clinic.

The social worker can offer a teaching service to her medical and nursing colleagues. If she is looked upon as a trusted member of the team, she will be able to initiate group discussion on the subject of abortion and be used as a colleague with whom staff on an individual basis will feel able to share their feelings about this emotive subject. She will be able, too, to ensure that her colleagues form a realistic picture of the difficulties which may confront the woman who wishes to continue with her pregnancy – for instance: inadequate financial resources, poor housing, lack of support from partner or family, or the sadness of deciding to have her baby adopted.

The benefits are threefold:

1. The social worker's role becomes better recognised and more highly valued.
2. Medical and nursing colleagues are encouraged to view the patient as a whole person.
3. The patient herself must inevitably benefit where she is

offered the expertise of a multidisciplinary team whose members are working in harmony rather than at cross purposes.

Although the work of the gynaecology and maternity social workers may appear highly specialised, the skills required in this area of work, the theoretical base employed in their approach and the insights gained have in fact much broader application to other patient groups. The ability to establish relationships quickly with people in crisis and to help them identify appropriate tasks and goals is obviously required of social workers in a wide variety of settings from work with women facing an unplanned pregnancy to work with people following a major crisis such as an air crash, flood, or rail disaster. The skilful use of informal support networks to complement statutory resources is demanded equally of the social worker in an area office, a paediatric ward, and a maternity or gynaecology hospital.

Finally, the concepts upon which the social work profession is based – notably the belief in client self-determination, human capacity for change and growth, and the client's right to be accepted as a person of human dignity and worth – are applicable whether the client group be women considering a termination of pregnancy, young adults in a unit for the severely physically disabled, in-patients on an acute psychiatric ward, or elderly people in a residential home.

Notes

1. Goffman, Erving, *Stigma: Notes on the management of spoiled identity*, Englewood Cliffs, NJ: Prentice Hall 1963.
2. Goffman, Erving, *Asylums*, Pelican, 1978.
3. Tuckett, David (ed.), *An Introduction to Medical Sociology*, London: Tavistock, 1986.
4. Parsons, T., *The Social System*, London: Routledge & Kegan Paul, 1951.
5. Phillips, M., and Dawson, J., *Doctors' Dilemmas: Medical ethics and contemporary science*, Brighton: Harvester, 1985.
6. Oakley, Ann, *The Captured Womb*, Oxford: Blackwell, 1986.
7. Kitzinger, Sheila, *The Midwife Challenge*, London: Pandora, 1988.
8. Association of Radical Midwives, *The Vision*, Association of Radical Midwives, 1986.
9. Ounsted, C., Roberts, J., Gordon, M., and Milligan, B., 'The fourth goal of perinatal medicine', *British Medical Journal*, 20 March 1982, pp. 879–82.
10. Hansell, Norris, *Person-in-distress: On the bio-social dynamics of adaptation*, New York: Human Scientific Press, 1977.

Suggestions for further reading

Black, J., and Holmes, J. 'Which mother knows best?', *Social Work Today*, **20**, 16, 15 December 1988, pp. 18–19.

Cowell, B., and Wainwright, D., *Behind the Blue Door*, London: Cassell, 1981.

Hannay, D., *Lecture Notes on Medical Sociology*, Oxford: Blackwell, 1988.

MacFarlane, A., and Mugford, M., *Birth Counts* London: HMSO, 1984.

Royal College of Midwives, *The Role and Education of the Future Midwife in the UK*, RCM, 1987.

Ruddock, R., *Roles and Relationships*, London: Routledge & Kegan Paul, 1976.

Sudnow, D. (ed.), *Studies in Social Interaction*, New York: Free Press, 1972.

Tuckett, D., and Kaufert, J. (eds), *Basic Readings in Medical Sociology*, London: Tavistock, 1978.

CHAPTER 7

Working with families from a different cultural background

ANABEL SHELLEY

Health professionals should concern themselves with race, ethnicity, religion and culture as much as with the age, gender and social class of their clients. Transcultural practice is awareness of the implications of communication between the health worker of one ethnic group and the client of another. These encounters should encompass an awareness of the physical, psychological and social aspects of care, of culture, religion and ethnicity together with an awareness of the political aspects of segregation and integration. British society consists of people with diverse national origins, cultural backgrounds and economic positions. Despite the ethnically pluralistic nature of our society, social work practice has not reflected this and fails in many instances to make available services which are appropriate to the specific needs of ethnic minorities.

Issues of race and culture are inextricably bound together and clearly understanding the boundaries and links between race and culture poses enormous difficulties for health and social services professionals. A high proportion of doctors are white and middle class with beliefs and values that reflect the ideology of the indigenous culture, and this unavoidably poses difficulties for the recipients of health care. The culture of the hospital can be a totally alien one even to a family which can understand language and procedures. For a family which has never learnt the language and customs of this country the experience will be frightening and bewildering. There may be a lack of understanding of religious and cultural customs among hospital staff, which will lead to the family feeling even more isolated. The social worker may be pressured by other professionals to make arrangements or seek resources that are inappropriate as time is not always available for adequate consultation with an interpreter. This is frequently due to the fact that hospital staff themselves are being pressed to deliver services where there are ever diminishing resources and serious underfunding. Social workers, whose focus is on the home and the community, can and should help ward and hospital staff to recognise racism and cultural insensitivity. There are customs, beliefs and rituals around death and illness that may be alien to them, but essential to families from different ethnic groups. These beliefs and customs need to be respected and adhered to. It is not proposed to examine in detail such rituals and customs as a detailed bibliography can be obtained from the Race Equality Unit at NISW.[1]

Racism expresses itself in a variety of ways, by denial in assuming that racism is non-existent and irrelevant, by claiming that racism is absent both in individual practice and the agency. Alternatively by intellectually acknowledging the racism but failing to acknowledge how this affects the family in their day-to-day living and experiences, therefore responding to their needs as if the family are a member of the indigenous culture. An example of this manifests itself in failing to provide interpreters for the family as a matter of course. Also within this context the way in which we deny colleagues from other ethnic groups their own experiences and perspectives. Racism is often perpetuated by placing the responsibility for anti-racist training and elimination of racism on black colleagues or by the practice of referring all black clients to a black worker, and the establishment of ethnic minority units, thereby pursuing apartheid in its most iniquitous form. Racism by adopting a colour-blind approach whereby ethnic minority clients are treated as white, which denies their specific experience as a member of a different ethnic group, ignoring the discrimination experienced by clients from other cultures in access to all welfare services, income status, health, housing and education. Racism by patronising clients by superficially acknowledging culture differences but the underlying assumption is maintained of the superiority of the indigenous culture. Racism through avoidance whereby an awareness of racism in social encounters and interactions with colleagues and the agency is accepted without confrontation or an expression of dissent.

The issue of cultural differences is examined in this chapter within a specialist setting, a multidisciplinary assessment centre for handicapped children. It looks at the experience of some of the families attending such a centre, and the work of the multidisciplinary team members. As parental values and opinions on child rearing are essentially culturally based, an awareness of cultural differences is particularly important in this setting. The family case studies are predominantly Asian; this is due to the fact that other ethnic groups are under-represented in the geographical area served by the assessment centre described. The word 'family' is used as a generic term to describe varieties of groupings of adults and children.

7.1   The assessment centre

In 1967 the Sheldon Report on the setting up of comprehensive assessment centres for handicapped children summarised the complex needs of children and parents:

Early identification, full assessment of disabilities and potentialities, prompt medical and surgical treatment, parent guidance, appropriate training and education, continuing support to the family and later, vocational training and placement in suitable employment or special care.[2]

The majority of children who attend such centres have evident multiple handicaps: physical, intellectual, social and behavioural difficulties. The major diagnostic category is cerebral palsy, and developmental delay. Many of the children have a number of mild and subtle difficulties which would be insignificant alone but combined constitute a definite handicap. The aim of the service is to support both families and professionals in their care of the handicapped child, make recommendations about educational needs, and to reduce parental anxiety and offer practical help. In many cases a variety of medical and community professionals are involved, and it is necessary to coordinate support to avoid duplication and stress for the families concerned. The reduction of anxiety can be achieved by a thorough discussion of diagnosis and causative factors, the medical aspects of prognosis, genetic counselling and a thorough evaluation of all aspects of the child's functioning. Parents are enabled to understand and acknowledge the outcome of the assessment through their own direct participation and observation of their child in different situations, noting that time has been taken to look carefully at all aspects and to see her in different moods.

In terms of practical help all aspects of daily living should be assessed, trying out equipment and suitable aids, toiletting, bathing, dressing, eating, drinking, sitting (chairs), mobility. The purpose being to build up parents' confidence in their own handling, demonstrating obliquely, through observation, or by specific instruction. Appropriate specific support should be arranged at home, i.e. physiotherapy, teacher/counsellor, social worker, home help, respite care and advice given to the playgroup/nursery/school which the child attends.

7.1.1   What does assessment mean to a family?

For many families the experience of undergoing the process of assessment is painful and stigmatising. It may be the first occasion in which they have had to acknowledge the difficulties facing their handicapped child and the implications this has for all the family. It may be the first comprehensive discussion of the child's diagnosis or, indeed, the poor prognosis for some children. This experience can be devastating for a family, especially in such a public setting with a group of professional staff.

The process of assessment, as experienced by the family, may appear to involve criticism of lifestyles, child-rearing practices and family function. Assessment is not a neutral process, and professionals bring to their work assumptions and values that more often than not reflect the dominant ideology that idealises family life, and ignores differences in class, race, income and gender.

The conditions in which children are brought up too often involve inadequate income with little or no access to resources that can relieve mothers of virtually total responsibility. Even when a man is part of the family women are seen, and see themselves, as being the person primarily responsible for child care.

Having a handicapped child adds to the usual requirements placed on women. In addition to providing day-to-day care, mothers are also mainly responsible for coping with out-patient appointments, visits to and from hospital during periods of stay which are a regular feature of many handicapped children's lives.[3]

The dominant ideology maintains that parenting is solely the personal and private responsibility of the family. The mother is seen as the person ultimately responsible for the nurture and well-being of the children, as well as other involved adults, husband and possibly her own and her husband's parents. As a result of this expectation, mothers are often the focus for criticism in child-rearing practices, and as such are expected to modify their behaviour accordingly. Middle-class parents are often seen as being over-demanding and over-ambitious for their children. Working-class parents may be seen as lacking in parenting skills and failing to stimulate their children adequately. Single parents are often seen as inadequate, the poverty of their circumstances rarely acknowledged. Parents from different cultures are often seen as unco-operative if they fail to take up or accept recommendations. Assessment can result in the stereotyping of families and their behaviour.

Inevitably the focus of stereotyping is often on race or cultural differences rather than the disability of the child. For some families the process of assessment can be a cathartic experience, allowing them to move closer to acknowledging their child's difficulties. The benefits of multidisciplinary assessment are often the effective coordination of community resources, physiotherapy, occupational therapy, social work support and respite care. Sometimes however, such a high level of community input can prove to be overwhelming for the family.

> *Case example*: Baby A. was referred to the centre for assessment, age 1 year. She is a profoundly handicapped little girl. The family are originally from Pakistan and have moved into the area recently. They live in a small county town, and are the only Pakistani family living on a pleasant housing estate on the outskirts of the town. Mr A. has just started his own business with one of his brothers. Mrs A. is at home with the children. She is a qualified teacher, but has not worked since the birth of Baby A. On visiting the family prior to assessment it was apparent that Mrs A. was extremely isolated and depressed. She did not know many of her neighbours and although now closer to her extended family, very much missed teaching and her social contacts through work. On assessment the team decided that Mrs A. needed more resources in order

to cope with Baby A. and a variety of professionals, a teacher/counsellor, a physiotherapist and a social worker were asked to visit the family at home.

Baby A. was followed up six months later at the centre, and in discussion with Mrs A. it emerged that although she valued the help and support she was being given, she had even less time to herself: almost every day of the week someone was visiting her at home and she felt quite overwhelmed and more unhappy. In discussion with other team members it was agreed that a more appropriate resource for Mrs A. was a childminder to enable her to get away from the family home for at least part of the day. She was keen to return to employment at least part time. The team's original view of Mrs A. was of a woman who was isolated and depressed. Her personal difficulties were not acknowledged and the perception of her needs distorted by seeing her as a passive Asian woman and homemaker. Her requirements were seen as being more input from community workers at home in order to help her cope, and alleviate her depression. It was only at review that it was agreed that the assessment of her needs was inaccurate and in need of re-evaluation.

Some families do not place the same value on assessment as the hospital staff involved in undertaking this task and this can be interpreted as not caring and bad parenting. If differences of race and culture also enter the picture, they confuse and blur the issues for both staff and the recipient family. They may also find this experience either painful or irrelevant and this is often not acknowledged by the professionals.

Case example: B. was referred to the centre for assessment, aged 3 years. She was delayed in her development with no language, unable to feed herself and still in nappies. She also had behaviour problems. Mrs D., her mother, was from a travelling community, separated from her husband and living with B. and her other children in two rooms in bed and breakfast accommodation. Mrs D. was very shy, and afraid of social workers. Her two eldest children had been taken into care and were living with foster families in another part of the country. She was very concerned and upset that her remaining children might be taken away from her, and that the assessment of B. might lead to a similar experience. The two eldest children who had been received into care were mentally handicapped. Despite transport having been arranged for the family, Mrs D. did not arrive on the first day of assessment. On the subsequent days B. attended with two of her teenage sisters, and on the final day Mrs D.'s sister attended the centre for a case conference to discuss the team's findings.

Some of the workers currently involved with the family were critical of Mrs D.'s behaviour, and documented a history of unattended hospital appointments and the family being out when agencies visited. Mrs D.'s fear of professionals and concerns about the possibility of losing her children were not acknowledged as a possible reason for her unwillingness to attend with B. She was seen as an inadequate and uncaring parent. Some of the assessment team's recommendations for B. were inappropriate. The recommendation for day-care for B. failed to acknowledge that this was culturally unacceptable to the family. Due to the family's inadequate accommodation, it would have been impossible for a physiotherapist visiting B. at home to be able to treat her, given the overcrowding and the family's circumstances. A recommendation, such as day-care for B., was also unacceptable to Mrs D. due to the beliefs of her travelling community. This particular community did not send their children to playgroups or childminders, children were not separated from their families until they attained school age. The issue of what help would have been appropriate for this family remained unresolved as they moved out of the area. However, it needs to be said that the family were not consulted as to what would have been acceptable to them in terms of support for B.

From these examples it is clear that professionals should avoid such stereotyping of women as mothers and carers as well as be aware of their own assumptions about family life and function. The individual's needs and cultural differences must always be acknowledged.

7.1.2   *Feelings are universal*

Human emotions are universal. Simon Olshansky in 'Chronic sorrow' describes the pervasive psychological reaction to the birth of a handicapped child as 'chronic sorrow'.[4] He argues this has not always been recognised by the agencies involved with the families. He describes in his paper parents' experiences throughout their lives and the life of the child, whether they continue to care for the child or she is placed in care. The intensity of this experience varies from person to person, situation to situation, family to family. Factors influencing the intensity of this experience, personality, ethnic group, religion and social class. Some families are able openly to show their grief, others find this more difficult, especially outside the family home. These feelings are shared amongst all families of children who would be considered handicapped in any society or cultural grouping. This may reflect assumptions that pathologise handicap and disability.

Professionals often become preoccupied with the notion of denial in families, particularly where they see the family as having difficulty in acknowledging their child's disability. A clear expression of grief is often treated as neurotic behaviour as opposed to a natural response to a tragedy. Family reactions include guilt, shame and anger and chronic sorrow. Despite these reactions families also derive satisfaction and happiness from the child's achievements. A family which has a disabled child is only too well aware that they and their children are often seen by society as inadequate or somehow as having failed as parents.

Diagnosis is a process and not a one-off event. Very often the only adults involved with a child, who can accept her problems are the medical staff in contact with the family. There is often an assumption made that a diagnosis of a child's disabilities and handicaps can be given in one interview. Some parents describe this experience as shocking, and the attitude they have met in staff as insensitive. Dr Alan Stein and Helen Woolley of Oxford University[5] have recently researched this process and made clear recommendations as to how this can be undertaken in a sensitive and caring way to enable the families' understanding. Families may deny the extent of a child's disability; difficulties vary, some move slowly and erratically towards acknowledgement, others become unnaturally optimistic about the child's potential. The regression of families needs to be recognised as a mechanism for coping with the pain of the reality of day-to-day living with the handicapped child. Workers often become impatient with families that behave in this manner, yet is it so bad that a family goes at its own pace in coping with the situation, particularly if the child is meeting their expectations in her own way? Most parents have a variety of experiences, good, bad, happy and sad in the bringing up of their children, however they can remain secure in the knowledge that eventually the child will achieve independence and be self-sufficient. Such a prospect is not a reality for the family with a handicapped child. They face an unrelenting dependency and constant demand, combined with a real concern for the child's future in the adult world, especially in the event of their own death.

How can families be helped by social workers and medical staff? In the first instance a notion of parental acceptance needs to be questioned. All families throughout the lives of their children whether they are without disability or handicapped, experience phases of acceptance and rejection at various times and in various situations. If we acknowledge this as normal, we need to review our own attitudes when dealing with families with a handicapped child. The majority of families do accept their child as handicapped and strive to meet that child's needs. However, to ask families to abandon their chronic sorrow is for the professionals to fail to acknowledge the endless frustrations of daily living with a handicapped child, the dependence and the relative lack of progress and change. Families in most instances have enormous courage and fortitude.

If the worker accepts that chronic sorrow is a normal response to an abnormal situation then families may be enabled to express their feelings more freely. The counselling and support of families is in some cases a lengthy process. In addition to the provision of information, families require the opportunity to express their feelings, and these feelings need to be acknowledged as appropriate. Some families need long-term counselling and support, for other families this opportunity is needed at various times throughout the life of their child. Families with handicapped children often have the need to discuss these feelings regularly. The need for repeated help is normal and should not be regarded as neurotic behaviour. It is perhaps necessary to consider that families need access to support and counselling as and when they feel they need it. The aim of counselling such families should be to enable them to acknowledge their own feelings as normal, as this will increase their ability to cope with the day to day living with their children.

7.2 Understanding the cultural background and how this affects approach and treatment

7.2.1 Stereotyping

Many social workers have expectations of how Asian parents view their mentally/physically handicapped child, which include various stereotypes:

1. The family will immediately reject the child on diagnosis.
2. The family will encounter feelings of resentment from other family members.
3. The family will feel stigmatised by the community.
4. The family will see the birth of a handicapped child as a punishment for their sins, or a test from God.
5. The birth of a handicapped child will provoke feelings of inadequacy especially for the mother.
6. The family will express embarrassment.
7. The family will fail to see the necessity to prepare for the future welfare of their child: God will protect him/her.
8. The Asian male is the dominant figure of the household and all communication should be made through him.[6]

The feelings experienced by families include profound guilt, confusion and disbelief, but families regardless of race experience these universal feelings. Families in the Asian community are very caring towards their children, as indeed most families in most societies are, and decisions about welfare are made by both parents. Some families do not wish to think of the future of their children without them as carers.

Religious belief may also be important, in that God can be seen as being the one and only director of the child's fate, and no one except him can change it. It is therefore important that a family is consulted before a programme of treatment is recommended, so that the medical staff can understand fully the family's feelings about such intervention. Families' knowledge of services and benefits can be poor: health visitors and social workers may fail to inform them of their entitlement. A service that is often not offered to an Asian family is respite care, due to some social workers' notion that short-term respite care is quite unacceptable to the Asian community, on the basis that such a service might imply the family are incapable and incompetent to look after their own child. Some families may well express this view, but such a negative attitude may be due to the social worker failing to explain clearly what short-term care or fostering involves. Inevitably families have reservations about using such a resource, and such a service would only be acceptable if the religious and cultural beliefs of the family were satisfied. Social services should actively promote the recruitment of foster families from all ethnic groups. The greatest difficulty faced by many families is communication and understanding. Social workers who are involved in the assessment of families and provision of services need to recognise and respect the cultural and religious requirements of these families and information of all services available should be produced in ethnic minority languages. (The Disability Alliance does publish *Benefits and Services for Disabled People* in Bengali, Gujerati, Hindi, Punjabi and Urdu.)

Cultural and religious needs should be a major focus of consideration if social services are to provide a service which is not only acceptable, but appropriate, in that it takes account of the religious and cultural element to ensure effective service delivery and better quality of health and social care for Asian families with handicapped children.[7] Services would need to ensure that all staff working with handicapped children and their families have anti-racist training, and this should be constantly reviewed to avoid stereotyping. Ethnic monitoring should be established to analyse service provision combined with the review of take up. More ethnic minority staff need to be recruited to undertake work with disabled children and adults. In the assessment of priorities, local authorities must take into account the needs of ethnic minorities. Specialist careers officers need to be made aware of the specific needs of ethnic minority children and young adults with disabilities. All local authorities should take up their responsibilities to provide adequate and appropriate service provision to ethnic minorities under the 1976 Race Relations Act. In many instances they have consistently failed to do so. It is also recommended that social workers should have access to interpreters to attend visits to the family. On many occasions interpreting is undertaken by the father, who may often only have basic English. There may be many questions and issues the family want to ask and discuss, and often these questions and issues remain unresolved as the lack of command of language restricts the family in expressing them. In some families members are not literate in either their mother tongue or English, therefore even if information is provided in mother-tongue leaflets, an interpreter and possibly a counsellor is essential if a meaningful and effective service is to be provided.

Case example: Mr and Mrs C. are a Pakistani family who have lived in the United Kingdom for about six years. Mr C. is unemployed due to severe rheumatoid arthritis. Baby C. was referred to the centre; his elder sister S. had previously been assessed due to problems with speech and mobility. Baby C. was showing signs of developing similar problems to his sister. The family arrived at the centre and it was immediately apparent that due to a significant deterioration in Mr C.'s arthritis he was scarcely able to walk. S. now 5, was only attending nursery part time, and it became apparent that she had slipped the net. Her educational needs had not been assessed and she had not started school. Mrs C. seemed depressed. The family's sole source of income was DSS Family Income Support. Their housing was poor and inadequately furnished.

During Baby C.'s assessment the doctor in charge was very concerned about Mr C., who was receiving treatment in a local hospital. He was a young man in his early 30s who had not seen an occupational therapist or been referred for rehabilitation. The assessment centre doctor expressed concern about Mr C. to the consultant rheumatologist who was currently managing his treatment, requesting a review of his medication, and also requesting a referral for rehabilitation. The consultant, on receiving the request immediately referred Mr C. to the social worker in his department on the basis that the problems were social in

origin. He informed the assessment centre doctor that Mr
C. was receiving appropriate medical treatment. Despite
a repeated request for a review and possible referral for
rehabilitation this was refused.

Although Mr C. spoke a little English, Mrs C. spoke
no English at all, and it was evident that the family
had difficulty in comprehending some aspects of the
assessment. An interpreter was only available for part
of the time of the family's attendance. Much of the
communication with the family was through Mr C. and
it was only through observation that members of the
team became concerned about Mrs C.'s emotional state.
The family's distress at having two handicapped children
became increasingly evident (this distress may well have
aggravated Mr C.'s symptoms), and their confusion about
resources for their children also became apparent.

At the end of the assessment the social worker who
had visited the family, referred them to the area team.
The referral listed the family's numerous difficulties and
requested counselling for them, in particular for Mrs C.
who, it was thought, was extremely vulnerable coping with
three members of her family suffering from disability. The
area team worker saw her own role as that of an adviser on
welfare rights. The social worker had to take a significant
amount of time and energy convincing area social work
colleagues of this family's emotional needs. Difficulties in
allocating a social worker to the family was due in effect
to lack of resources in the present climate of cutbacks and
underfunding.

Social workers are influenced by their own cultural conditioning. The cultural differences in shared assumptions and
prescriptive rules often lead to incongruent messages being
given to a family from a different culture. Some recurrent
areas of difficulty in work with ethnic families include the role
of culture-bound symptoms and family structures that do not
conform to the prescribed norms of the dominant culture. Social
workers working with families with different cultural norms
will be tempted to restructure the 'deviant' families along lines
reflecting their own cultural ideals. Family problems are therefore
often viewed from a white Western ethnocentric position. We

handle phenomena from other cultures, using concepts and ideas derived from our own cultural background. Some of the current ethical and practice training of social workers maintains a view that the British population is integrated and that racial factors are insignificant, and if the practice of universality is pursued, this will ensure equality amongst individuals.

Such fundamental misunderstanding of black people's experience and the failure of white social workers to appreciate the power and privilege they enjoy because they live in a racist society facilitates their fostering racist stereotypes in their practice.[8]

The traditional case work model relies heavily on the individualisation of client problems, denying the social and political context within which the individual finds herself. The failure to acknowledge contextual issues offers the client an approach from a different cultural group which at best is inappropriate and at worst woefully inadequate.

7.2.2   Problems of interpretation

A practice which has become widespread is managing without an interpreter during the assessment phase of social work with the family. Interpreters are frequently not available, and it can be a difficult and lengthy process to find a person with a good command of language in both the mother tongue of the family and English. As a result social workers often make do with simplified English and even sign language, or by relying on other members of the family themselves to undertake this task. There is however a growing awareness amongst local authorities of the need to provide their clients from different ethnic groups with competent trained interpreters in order to provide an accessible and appropriate service.

Social workers who work closely with medical colleagues in a multidisciplinary setting need to be aware that often colleagues' training as well as their own in anti-racist practice is either non-existent or minimal, therefore often the role of the social worker in such a setting is to raise awareness as to different cultural and religious beliefs, and different practices in child rearing. This will often entail dealing with blatant racism, and judgemental and inappropriate comments on family lifestyle. As a social worker the role of advocacy in this area of practice is often difficult and potentially confrontational, requiring that the social worker needs to use all her skills in negotiation to avoid further alienation of clients.

Case example: G. is Mr and Mrs N.'s eldest son, aged 10 years. He has exhibited behavioural problems at school, and is now significantly behind in his class. He was diagnosed prior to attending primary school as being mildly developmentally delayed. Mr and Mr N. are originally from Pakistan and live in a small street in the city centre. They were re-housed fairly recently due to persistent racial harassment which culminated in racial attacks on the family home. Mr N.'s brother had his family live next door, also re-housed for the same reason. On visiting the family an interpreter accompanied the social worker, as Mrs N. did not speak any English. This initial visit lasted about two hours and was particularly distressing for Mrs N. as she said she was very upset about G. and his difficulties, particularly as he was their eldest son. A significant part of the interview was spent in explaining to Mrs N. the purpose of assessment, including the more difficult task of preparing the family for the fact that there might possibly be no diagnosis or remedy for G.'s problems. Throughout G.'s attendance for assessment his mother was present: his father was only able to attend for part of his assessment, and this was only arranged after numerous telephone calls by the doctor in charge to the factory where Mr N. worked. The need for Mr N. to attend was due to the fact that an interpreter was only available for two short periods throughout the week. As a result of Mr N. attending, his pay was cut, and again it took several telephone calls and letters from medical staff and the social worker to reinstate his lost pay. The whole experience of assessment was very painful and distressing for the family, and the medical team had enormous difficulties in communicating with the family, not just due to language differences, but due to the family's lack of understanding of G.'s limitations, and the fact that there was no remedy available. Many families, irrespective of race, experience this same difficulty. The follow-up visit to the family at home was made by the assessment centre social worker accompanied by a Pakistani social worker who already knew the family. The assessment centre social worker was concerned that the family be offered counselling and support in order to help them acknowledge G.'s needs and difficulties. Co-visiting with an Asian social worker enabled the assessment team worker to seek the appropriate resource that would also be acceptable to the family.

Some members of the team were critical of Mr and Mrs N.'s parenting, and the social worker had to take immense care in advising them about different child-rearing practices. This was necessary in order for the team to consider carefully the advice they gave to the family in respect of G.'s behavioural problems.

Apart from the need to use an interpreter and finding an interpreter who is available, arranging a visit that is convenient to the family can often take up a significant amount of time. A visit to the family can also take considerably longer than a straightforward interview, where there are no language or cultural differences. Given these difficulties, it is important that social workers report these problems to their agencies, and be firm in their resolve where there is a need to undertake an interview with an interpreter present in order that they might be appropriate to a family's needs.

Where the majority of staff are white, there is a clear need for a comprehensive interpreting service. Interpreters can act as intermediaries between the agency and the community. The recruitment and training of interpreters should be seen as an overall review of the relationship between staffing and service delivery. Social workers should insist that all interviews undertaken with families from a different ethnic grouping with a different language should be done with the aid of an interpreter and encourage their departments to provide this service. Some research on this subject has been undertaken by the NISW Race Equality Unit.

7.3 Child protection: Facing contentious issues

In recent years society and social workers have become more aware of the numbers of children subjected to abuse. Low birth-weight babies and handicapped children are at risk because care is so stressful physically, emotionally and financially for their carers. There are essentially two groups of abused, handicapped children: those born disabled who are being abused, and those who were not born with a disability, but become so through abuse or injury.

White social workers working with black families when issues of statutory responsibility arise are often fearful of being assertive from the fear of being seen as racist. This was evident in the case of Jasmine Beckford, and in *A Child in Trust*, the issue of race is scarcely mentioned.[9] The fact that the family social worker was white and might have encountered both professional and personal difficulties in relating to the family is never mentioned. The social workers involved with this family may well have been very fearful about being seen as racist, and possibly as a result of this, did not tackle some of the child care issues more vigorously. There is no mention in the report that this may well have influenced the decision-making of the social workers involved. The only recommendation referring to race refers to placements for children.

The greater effort should be made to recruit black families as prospective foster parents in order to provide the greatest measure of choice to local authorities for fostering or adopting black children in their care.[10]

If workers cannot address race directly, how can they offer an effective service to their clients from other cultures, and if they are unable to face the issue themselves, how can they undertake child protection work without failing to protect the vulnerable child?

If practice with families is influenced by the use of traditional case work methods, this can be a barrier to confronting racist practice. It is easy to see the black client/white worker relationship as separate from wider political issues. The case-work model encourages social workers to treat prejudice and discrimination as individual pathology. White social workers undertaking child protection work with clients from ethnic minorities must be prepared to make a detailed study of their clients' cultural background and value system, including an understanding of habits, family structures, religion, education, and the role of men and women in the family.

Child abuse procedures rarely take cultural or physical differences into account, adopting a colour-blind approach. *Protecting Children* states:

although no culture sanctions extreme harm to a child cultural variations in child care patterns exist. A balanced assessment must incorporate a cultural perspective, but guard against being over sensitive to cultural issues at the expense of promoting the safety and well being of the child, e.g. in deciding who will undertake the assessment consideration should be given to the possibility of allocating a worker from the same cultural background as the family, or co-working with an individual who can assist the social worker in understanding the cultural issues, or where appropriate, to involving a language interpreter – above all it is important that social workers should feel comfortable about raising cultural issues with children or families proactively.[11]

If child protection work is to be undertaken effectively, social workers need anti-racist training and support through interpreting services. The agency needs to be committed to anti-racist practice with some access to appropriate information services and possibly social work colleagues who either themselves are from ethnic minorities, or have experience in working with families from other cultures. Social workers undertaking child protection work should be committed to challenge their own racism and the racism of their agency if they are to be effective in their practice.

> *Case example*: S., aged 5 years, was referred for assessment. The school had expressed concern about her level of developmental delay. She was attending a mainstream primary school. S. is the fourth child of Mr and Mrs G.. The family are originally from India, and have only a few members of the extended family living locally. The social worker visited the family with an interpreter as the health visitor reported the mother's knowledge of English was limited. Mr G. is a factory worker and the family live in a small house in the poorer part of the city. Mr G. did not attend the centre during the week, although he came for the case discussion at the end of the assessment.
>
> The team became increasingly concerned during the assessment about Mrs G.'s lack of understanding of S.'s

significant degree of mental handicap and her openly hostile manner when handling S. The psychologist was extremely worried about S. and her relationship with her mother, and expressed this concern openly at the case discussion. Due to the worries expressed by the assessment team, community agencies involved with the family at that point openly discussed their anxieties and disclosed a series of incidents reported by neighbours of neglect and possible abuse. None of the community agencies had referred the family to social services despite the fact that there had been a high level of awareness at the possibility of neglect and abuse. The family were immediately referred to the local social services department, and were shortly visited by a duty social worker, the assessment centre social worker and an interpreter.

In the case discussion it became apparent that the community agencies were reluctant to believe the allegations made about the family, they were unanimously fearful of being seen as racist, and thinking that they were failing to understand cultural differences in child-rearing practices. The family were allocated a social worker to help them to understand S.'s difficulties and prevent further neglect.

7.4   Anti-racist training

Practising social workers frequently do not have access to anti-racist training. Social work students often come on placement with little or no understanding of race or culture. It therefore would seem essential to consider what are the training needs of both practitioners and social work students.

If social work is to address the issue of racism and cultural oppression, the development of anti-racist practice is essential. Social workers whose agency deals with clients from different ethnic cultures must address personal and political issues, so that, by addressing these very difficult issues, they can be incorporated into mainstream practice. CQSW courses themselves must also develop practice to meet the needs of different ethnic groups.

Social work, redefined according to anti-racist criteria, is not about social control, but about realising significant improvement in the life chances and well-being of individuals, regardless of their gender, race, class, age, physical or intellectual abilities, sexual orientation, religious affiliation or linguistic capability. Anti-racist social work, therefore, is a bridge between social work in a racist society and social work in a non-racist one.[12]

Initially social workers have to tackle their own racism by actively seeking to improve awareness of racism in themselves and in their colleagues. Skin colour and culture determine experience. Social workers need to examine how their own attitudes and behaviour contribute to racism, and if they can address this in themselves openly they can avoid self-blame and guilt. Racism is learnt through social conditioning, and is not inborn. Social workers need to examine the use of personal terms and phrases that might be seen by others as degrading and hurtful, and to disagree openly with racist jokes and actions. They have to take active steps to become more knowledgeable about other cultures, lifestyles, values and histories, and in so doing in work with colleagues who are from different cultures they need to accept and value their contribution to practice. In practice and within the agency they need to campaign for equality of opportunity and to avoid making uninformed judgements about different cultural norms. They need to maintain a standard of assessment based on individual needs and avoid cultural stereotyping. Individual needs will vary and there has to be an awareness of issues such as isolation, support and community.

The Social Care Association has defined dimensions of crucial importance in working with families:

1. The emphasising of credibility of black norms and lifestyles.
2. Measures taken to remedy inequalities in policies, procedures and practice.
3. Where appropriate, the talking through of emotional and cultural conflicts.
4. The respecting of cultural identities and the understanding of the nature of different cultural heritages.
5. The enabling of groups to take pride in their cultural identity.
6. The meeting of the needs of a person as relevant to that individual.
7. The tackling of racism (wherever and whenever it occurs) with dignity, self-respect and self-assertiveness.

8. The support and encouragement of black people in their exercising of their leadership skills.
9. The understanding of the effects of racism on black people, e.g. isolation of the individual, lack of personal worth, loss of personal dignity and feelings of powerlessness.[13]

7.4.1   Training needs

Communication between social workers and families of a different race or culture is at best fraught with difficulties. If the social worker and the family do not share a common language then the problem is compounded. Social workers and interpreters need to be trained to work with each other.

Pathway[14] believes that in training for social workers, working with interpreters is an essential concomitant of training for the interpreters themselves. This helps to resolve ethical issues such as the following:

1. How far does responsibility for ensuring effective communication rest with the social worker and how far with the interpreter?
2. Does the client have the right to an interpreter, or is it at the discretion of the social worker?
3. What if the client refuses an interpreter, but the social worker is not confident that effective communication will take place without one?
4. Is it all right for an interpreter to interpret for clients with whom she does not share a first language?

Training enables social workers to understand the dynamics of an interpreted interview and the ways in which the social worker can help – or hinder the interpreting process. Pathway's in-service course focuses on skills such as the following:

1. Briefing the interpreter effectively.
2. Creating a relationship with the client, too, and apart from the interpreter.
3. Controlling your own communication in terms of quantity, complexity or thought and language and style of delivery in such a way as to be as helpful as possible to the interpreter.

4. Maintaining control of the interview while allowing inter-preter interventions where appropriate.
5. Using constructively the 'thinking space' generated in an interpreted interview as a result of the slow pace.

The course is aimed to develop trust and respect between social worker and interpreter. In particular, Pathway is anxious to dispel the frequent misconception that 'if you can speak two languages, you can interpret'. Interpreting is a complex skill. If the social worker undervalues it the working relationship will be undermined and the client will get a less effective service. If anti-racist training is to be addressed at all levels then CQSW courses must provide anti-racist training for students. This issue was raised by Juliet Edmunds and Diana Powell, social work educators who published a paper in 1980, 'Multi-racial social work', in which they wrote about their work with social work students during which they had provided in-depth training on race and social work practice. They argue that such training should be a compulsory element of CQSW courses. They gave considerable thought to their roles as white trainers and share a fundamental belief that undertaking race awareness training is central to tackling racism. They have adopted the practice of seeing black students prior to the start of the racism awareness programme, asking them if they wish to participate. They are not willing to collude with students who take the view of race being a black problem, and having thus defined the issue then expect black students to be both conscience and scapegoat as and when the issue arises. They are also aware that offering black students the choice of participating in the programme is no choice, if they opt out, they are copping out, therefore further complicating their already difficult relationship with the dominant group:

Being acknowledged a resource person alongside the trainers is problematic as it serves to highlight black differences, and can increase pressure on black students to identify racism and also to suggest remedies.[15]

In the group Juliet Edmunds and Diana Powell managed to highlight some of the less overt manifestations of racism. White colleagues often react with considerable anxiety to any suggestion their attitudes might be insensitive and unhelpful to black people. This can inevitably lead to tension and conflict within a group setting. Because of the dynamics of white racism in social work education both trainers have become increasingly aware of the need for good support for students during training and afterwards in their agency settings.

7.4.2 Practice needs

Social workers need to familiarise themselves with good practice, as used by some of their colleagues in the community. In terms of social work practice, Old Trafford Social Services are attempting to counteract the racism experienced by their clients; the team won second prize in the 'Equal Opportunities Section' of the *Social Work Today* awards.

The five-member team are themselves multi-racial, and their aim is to provide a service to the multi-racial community that is ethnically sensitive. Team recruitment was on the basis of specialist knowledge and skills in order to make closer links with the local multi-racial community. The majority of the funding for the team comes from central government Section 11 funding; specific criterion for such a resource is that services are developed that are appropriate for ethnic minority groups. June Manning, team leader, states:

Child protection is a very complex issue, most social work theory and training is white, middle class and male based. There is a way of dealing with cultural issues which impinge on child protection – so we work jointly, i.e. a black worker and a white worker together, on an equal basis to offer advice and information.[16]

An important development since the team was established has been the setting up of a black workers' group. The aim of this group is to offer both professional and personal support, to help reduce experiences and feelings of isolation. The group also has an educative role for members, clients and social services. Black social worker Allan Simpson is satisfied that the presence of three black social workers on the team is not just tokenism, and that as a result of this people are more assertive. June Manning admitted to feeling vulnerable initially as a white team manager; she delegated a lot of her tasks to black workers in order to learn from them. She believes this is necessary if social work as a profession is to recognise that experience is as valid as academic achievement.

Notes

1. See suggestions for further reading for address.
2. *Child Welfare Centres*, (The Sheldon Report), London: HMSO, 1967.
3. Hanmer, J., and Statham, D., *Women and Social Work: Towards a woman-centred practice*, BASW, 1988, p. 54.
4. Olshansky, Simon, in: *Social Work With Families*, E. Younghusband (ed.), London: Allen & Unwin, 1975 (first published 1965).
5. Woolley, H., Stein A., Forrest, G. C., and Baum, J. D., in: *The Care of the Child with Life-threatening Disease*, 1989. See chapter entitled 'The Helen House studies: An analysis of hospice care for children'.
6. Shah, R., *Attitudes, Stereotypes and Service Provision and the Asian Client with Mental/Physical Handicap*, Manchester Council for Community Relations, 1987.
7. *ibid*.
8. *ibid*. It should be pointed out here that CCETSW has set out new guidelines for a DipSW, incorporating training in race and gender issues.
9. Blom-Cooper, L., *A Child in Trust*, report of the panel of inquiry into the circumstances surrounding the death of Jasmine Beckford, London Borough of Brent, 1985.
10. *ibid*.
11. *Protecting Children: A guide for social workers undertaking a comprehensive assessment*, London: HMSO, 1988.
12. Dominelli, Lena, *Anti-Racist Social Work*, BASW, 1989.
13. Social Care Association, 'Anti-racist practice'. The social care practice committee reports further on ways of tackling racism in social care, *Social Work Today*, 4 June 1988.
14. Pathway is a small industrial unit based in a college of further education in the London Borough of Ealing.
15. Edmunds, Juliet, and Powell, Diana, 'Are You Racist Too?' *Community Care*, September 1985.
16. Wilson, Melba, 'Equal service for a multiracial community', *Social Work Today*, 6 July 1989.

Suggestions for further reading

Bryan, B., Dadzie, S., and Scafe, S., The Heart and The Race: Black Women's Lives in Britain, London: Virago, 1985.

Cheetham, J., Hames, W., Loney, M., Mayh, B., and Prescott, W. (eds), *Social and Community Work in a Multi-Racial Society*, London: Harper & Row, 1981.

Fryor, P., *Staying Power: The history of black people in Britain*, London: Pluto, 1984.

Race Equality Unit publications available from:
National Institute for Social Work (NISW),
5/7 Tavistock Place,
London
WC1H 9SS
Ask for bibliography.

CHAPTER 8

Hospital and the child

MARDI CHANDLER, ROSEMARY CLARIDGE
and JENNY LEE

The admission of a child to hospital is now considered to be less traumatic than twenty years ago when ward routine was sacrosanct, Sister's word was law, and parents as visitors were scarcely tolerated. Nowadays the paediatric ward or out-patient department belies much of the sorrow and pain which families are experiencing. The wards are bright, the children are often not in bed but in the playroom, toys abound, and parents are often resident with their children.

The work of paediatric social workers is as varied as the families with whom they come into contact. This chapter will focus on just a few aspects of the work undertaken, in an attempt to illustrate the enormous variety of work and the extent of the challenge in a typical paediatric setting.

First discussed are families facing chronic handicap and illness, child protection and bereavement counselling. Then will be considered working with families in crisis, and finally the child in the out-patient clinic.

A large percentage of the social worker's case-load will be made up of children who are suffering from life-threatening and/or chronic illness and children who are profoundly handicapped, either mentally, physically, or both. The first contact parents may have with the social services department is when they meet the social worker in the hospital. This introduction is of vital importance and will set the scene for the months and years to follow. Their fears and prejudices with regard to social work can be confirmed or dispelled with this first contact. The point of entry may be extremely difficult – when parents have just been told that their child has a devastating diagnosis which may lead to death, to a life of chronic illness, or crippling handicap, it may seem like the final insult to then have to meet a social worker who is going to ask them how they feel. Anger and denial are common in these early stages. Contact can be facilitated by an early offer of practical support – be it financial, help with child care arrangements, help at home, linking with community services, or liasing with the DSS.

8.1 Chronic illness and handicap

Case example: a chronically ill child Christopher was 2 when the social worker first met his parents. He had been diagnosed as having cystic fibrosis.[1] His older brother Neville had died of the same condition the previous year, during which time the family had been well supported by another social worker. However they were always very private and reluctant to talk about their feelings. In some ways Christopher's arrival had helped the family through the worst days of Neville's final illness and it could be argued that they had still not properly mourned him. When the new social worker first met Rob and Jean, Christopher's parents, they had just been told that Christopher had an inoperable heart condition and that it was unlikely that he would live longer than twelve months.

There seemed little a social worker could do, other than acknowledge and share their pain, encourage them to talk about Neville, and help them find some of the coping mechanisms which they had learned during Neville's illness and death. A practical role was all they would allow the social worker at that stage. Jean could not drive and welcomed transport being arranged for her. Money at times was tight and help with travelling expenses was gratefully accepted. Robert's job was under threat and intervention with his boss helped him understand why Robert had to take so much time off work. A year later Christopher was admitted in the terminal stages of his illness. Jean could only allow herself to face up to what was happening for short periods. In between she would allow her hopes to rise as Christopher responded briefly to a new drug. Each time his condition deteriorated it was as if it were entirely unexpected. Robert remained strong and supportive, using the social worker to express his grief, to weep in private in order to be strong for Jean.

It was of vital importance that any discussions which the medical staff had with the parents included the social worker. In this way the social worker was fully aware of Christopher's continuing critical condition (in spite of Jean's optimism), and was there to help the parents express and understand their feelings as the medical situation and plans changed from day to day.

Christopher's final illness was long and drawn out, which allowed his parents to make plans for his terminal care. The social worker remained in contact with the family for several years after his death. As with Neville the family found it hard to grieve, but when the social worker visited they used the time with her to do some grief work, after which they made enormous efforts to reconstruct their lives and to try to look forward to a future without children.

Mourning does not simply involve grieving for a loved one who has died. It also includes grieving for the healthy child one did not have, for all the hope and future that are denied. Christopher's parents not only had to grieve two children who died but had also suffered years of anticipatory mourning in an effort to prepare themselves for their certain loss.

Case example: a child with profound handicap Sammy's parents grieved for the child they did not have, and although he was still alive that process helped them to detach themselves from him. Sammy was 4 years old and suffered from the most extreme form of mental and physical handicap. He was born very prematurely and for many weeks his life hung in the balance. When they eventually took him home his parents allowed themselves some guarded optimism with regard to his future. Sadly, as the months went by it became increasingly apparent that Sammy was going to be a very handicapped little boy who probably would not live for very many years. When Sammy was 3 his mother became pregnant with twins. They too were born prematurely but fortunately had an easier neonatal period, and were normal. The social worker first met the mother, Janice, when the twins were discharged from the neonatal unit. Sammy, who had been cared for by a relief foster mother, was returned home and not surprisingly Janice found she could not cope. Although Janice had been receiving help from the local social services department it seemed that it had not been possible to fully appraise the needs of the whole family before the twins' birth. In planning a package of care the following important factors had to be recognised:

1. Sammy was dependent for all care – feeding him was very difficult and time-consuming and he could scream for hours on end for no apparent reason. He also slept poorly at night.
2. The twins, being premature, needed two-hourly feeds day and night, which continued for some considerable time until they had caught up on their weights.
3. Janice was exhausted having had a Caesarean section, having worried about possible damage to the twins because of their prematurity, and having spent some weeks making fairly lengthy trips to the hospital and to visit Sammy in care.
4. Charles, her husband, had recently started a new job following a period of unemployment. He felt he could not afford to jeopardise his employment by asking for any time off.
5. Janice could not set foot out of the house as she had no way of transporting three children safely in the car and could not manage to push three children in prams unaided.

The task of the social worker was to try to seek some practical solutions to these problems as it seemed clear that with such pressure on the mother her relationship with the children was going to suffer, and the marriage could also be jeopardised. A case conference was convened involving all the professionals concerned. It was then agreed that relief care of Sammy would continue on several nights per week. The foster mother would also have the twins one night per week to allow the parents an unbroken night's sleep and the chance to go out together. Home help would be granted and volunteers from a local independent mental handicap unit would come each afternoon to care for the twins to allow Janice to spend time with Sammy.

Over the following year concern increased with regard to the parents' ability to care for Sammy. As their twins grew and developed normally, so Janice and Charles began to appreciate for the first time just how handicapped Sammy was, how abnormal he looked, and how he prevented them from doing many normal family things. On one occasion Sammy was admitted to hospital with bruising. In an interview with the paediatrician and the social worker the parents were 'given permission' to say they had had enough. They were praised for doing such a wonderful job in caring for Sammy, but were encouraged to put the needs of their healthy children first. After much anguish and soul searching they were eventually able to relinquish Sammy into care, although they remained in regular contact with him.

Janice and Charles had always been viewed as model parents of a handicapped child. They had made the initial adjustment to caring for a handicapped child and had always believed that they would be Sammy's principal carers. However, situations change, needs vary, and feelings alter. With help they came to realise that they did not want to devote the rest of their lives to care for such a severely handicapped child. Fortunately, a sufficiently good relationship had been built up with both the social worker and the paediatric consultant for Janice to honestly state how she felt and for work to be done with both parents to help them relinquish Sammy, to concentrate on the marital relationship and on their relationship with the twins.

In this instance it was to the parents' advantage to have two social workers. The hospital social worker could see where the strains lay for the family and could liaise with the area team social worker who had been viewing the situation simply from the needs of the handicapped child.

The parents had felt reluctant to voice any complaints to the local team for fear they might lose the existing support services. When Sammy was finally admitted with bruising, instead of invoking the whole child protection machinery it was agreed that the most supportive line of action would be to allow the parents to make the decision themselves. They could see that Sammy's needs would be better met by his foster mother, with whom both he and they had a very comfortable relationship.

Working in tandem with colleagues in the area teams is not always easy. Each social worker can have a different perspective on the family and the family, in turn, can use this situation manipulatively. Here the relationship between the two social workers concerned was, at first, strained. It was only with repeated and regular contact between the two teams that sufficient trust was developed for the social workers to understand that the parents did 'split', that is give different and sometimes conflicting information to each worker. Like a marriage, the professional relationship with a colleague also has to be worked at!

8.2 Life-threatening illness

Case example: a child with cancer Zoe was 12 when she was diagnosed as having an osteosarcoma (malignant tumour of the bone). Her parents were immediately informed that she had cancer, that she would have to have her leg amputated, that her chances of survival were less than 50 per cent, and that if the cancer did not kill her there was a chance that the chemotherapy might. They were also warned not to share this information with the daughter and not to inform any of their relatives for fear that they, in turn, might tell her. Initially Zoe was treated at the orthopaedic hospital but was transferred for chemotherapy to the children's ward of the district general hospital, where the paediatric staff strongly disagreed with the orthopaedic surgeon's unwillingness to tell the child of her diagnosis. The social worker, who was based at the orthopaedic hospital, was faced with the conflict of defying the consultant's wishes or failing in her duty to the family. She could not convince the surgeon that it was important to be open with Zoe so as to allow her time to prepare herself for the prospect of amputation. The parents were distraught. The only time they could express their true feelings was with the social worker and the paediatric staff in the general hospital. The remainder of the time they had to put on an act with their son, with Zoe herself, with friends and relatives. Fortunately they were to meet a determined young paediatric registrar who did not feel in any way duty bound to follow the wishes of the surgeon. He strongly advised the parents to tell Zoe what was going to happen, but before they had the chance to do this Zoe took the matter into her own hands. That night Zoe said to her mother, 'I have cancer, don't I? I'm going to lose my leg like Michael' (another child on the ward who had undergone amputation). Her mother was able to answer her truthfully and the work with Zoe could begin. Fortunately the surgeon was able to accept that it was in the child's best interest to be told about her illness by a well-intentioned paediatrician and was finally relieved of the obligation to tell her himself.

Initially Zoe adopted a very pragmatic approach – if losing her leg meant that she would not die then she would willingly face amputation. She survived surgery with humour, making jokes at her own expense. Post-operatively she held court in her cubicle, playing the fool, acting as if she had no cares in the world. By the time she was ready to recommence chemotheraphy, following surgery, she was a changed child. She became mute, she tore at her fingers till they bled, she wept, she snapped at her poor heartbroken mother whenever she tried to comfort her. And when she finally lost her hair Zoe refused to be seen in the outside world. The social worker spent hours with the family, trying to help them understand Zoe's behaviour. Zoe had not been given sufficient time to prepare herself for amputation, had coped by denial when facing surgery, and was now forced to face life without a leg, without hair, and was also having to face the prospect of death.

Over the weeks and months the social worker spent time with Zoe on her own, talking, reading, encouraging her to draw, to paint, to sew, to concentrate on all her exceptional talents. The reward at the end would be to meet her favourite pop star. When her hair had just begun to grow back Zoe felt the time was right. With her brother and her best friend she went to have afternoon tea in a smart London hotel with her idol. The girl who had been unable so much as to set foot in the outside world even appeared on television! Three years later Zoe was a bouncy 16-year old, bright at school, and popular with the boys. She did not like anyone to talk about her artificial limb and always wore trousers. She was determined that being an amputee would not prevent her from leading a full and active life.

The difficulties of working in a secondary setting are highlighted when the social worker and family are in conflict with the opinion of the consultant who is treating the child. Accordingly it can be very hard to provide the support a family may need while continuing to help them retain confidence in the treatment their child is receiving. As an employee of the local authority the hospital social worker has contact with any patient or relative with the 'permission' of the consultant medical staff. To differ from the views of the consultant may lead to a mutual lack of trust which could endanger the working relationship.

8.3 Group work with parents

Most of the work which the paediatric social worker does is with individual children and their families, but it can also be very useful to work with groups of children or parents of children who have the same condition. A very special skill is involved in helping children or parents cope with the different stages of their illness and learn how to protect themselves when hearing how much better (or worse) someone else may be doing. This cannot be highlighted more poignantly than with a group of parents of children with cancer. At any one time, attending such a group there may be the parent of a child who has just been diagnosed, a parent of a child who is experiencing distressing and alarming complications of treatment, and a parent of a child who has died. Of course it may be true to say that many of these parents self-select: if they do not wish to expose themselves to the sometimes painful information they may receive in the group, they will not attend. Much initial work must be done to prepare parents prior to attendance at the group. Often, following each meeting, individual work will have to be undertaken with group members, helping them to understand why some parents have behaved in a particular way, acknowledging which areas may have been especially painful for them and which they may have been trying to avoid, such as the possible death of their child. These disadvantages are far outweighed by the friendship, consolation, and support offered by the other group members. The children too find great comfort in learning that they are not the only ones who are suffering from such an appalling illness; they learn to encourage each other and gradually the older ones learn to face up to the prospect of dying, or of their friends dying.

8.4 Bereavement counselling

Working in a large regional hospital with a university department and a world-renowned neonatal unit means carrying a heavy case-load of children with rare, serious, and life-threatening illnesses. This also means that a significant proportion of parents who are referred to the social worker have children who die. Bereavement counselling forms a large proportion of her work. Studies have shown that it takes at least two years following the death of an adult to complete the grieving process[2]. With children it takes much longer and it can be argued that the process is never finished. It is unnatural to survive one's children and in this age it is rare. Most Victorians expected to bury two or three of their children. Today's parents plan their small families carefully and expect all of their children to survive. For many parents the death of their child is the first death they have ever experienced. They may never have attended a funeral before; they may not know what is expected of them; they wonder if they are being morbid in wanting to hold their dead child; they do not know if they are allowed to plan their own style of funeral or if they must follow some rules.

It is much easier to undertake bereavement counselling with

a family previously known to the social worker. This forms a very strong argument for meeting a family with a child with a life-threatening illness at an early stage in diagnosis. There are no rules for grieving. Parents, brothers, and sisters will grieve at their own pace in their own time. Grieving is a natural process and does not need the help of the professional to facilitate it. However, monitoring the situation by providing continuing support will allow the social worker to assess how the family is proceeding with their grief work and whether they are encountering any particular difficulties. This can be an especially stressful time for a marriage and for the relationships with surviving children. Some parents try to deny their grief for fear of sinking into an abyss out of which they may never crawl. Others can only express their feelings of grief and cannot pick up the pieces of what is left of their lives. All of these phases are part of the normal pattern of grief, but if they become too lengthy, if people become stuck in them and cannot progress to the next phase, we can see this as an abnormal grief reaction and one which will probably need some professional intervention. This could mean working with the whole family for some sessions, referral to the psychiatric services, or providing more intensive help for the individual family member concerned.

8.5 Child protection

When a child is suspected of being physically abused she is usually referred for a paediatric opinion. If the paediatrician feels that the child's injuries have been caused non-accidentally, or if she is unsure about the account given, the child will be admitted to hospital and the paediatric social worker informed. The task of the hospital social worker is to collate whatever information is necessary to help all the professionals concerned come to a decision as to what action, if any, is necessary to protect the child. This will involve checking if the child's name is on the Child Protection Register and if the family is known to the local social work office, discussing the situation with the health visitor (if under school age) or with the school (if over 5), with the GP, or with any other professionals concerned. A detailed history will be taken from the parents, or suspected perpetrators, and a case conference convened. Most parents/caretakers are incensed at being accused of deliberately injuring their child; therefore one of the first emotions the social worker encounters is anger. Many parents fear that their child will be removed from them and therefore feel they must deny what has happened at all costs. We know there are many warning factors which may predispose a family to abuse a child.[3] However, we also know that child abuse is not confined to the most socially disadvantaged groups. The social worker must remain entirely neutral; she can only listen to what all the parties involved have to say, to note the discrepancies in the accounts given, to invite explanations of these discrepancies, and to present all the relevant information to the case conference.[4]

Children who are the subject of case conferences may not necessarily have been *physically* abused; they may have been neglected, emotionally deprived, their development avoidably impaired, or have been sexually abused.

Case example: a physically abused child Tamsin was a 6-month-old twin with a fractured femur. Her parents were enraged that anyone could think that they could injure their own child. The father insisted that he had been playing with the baby's legs when he heard a loud crack. They immediately sought medical attention and kept insisting that had they themselves injured their child they would not have taken her to the doctor. They were angry with the social worker for failing to accept their account and were resentful that Tamara, the other twin, was also admitted to the ward. They saw the area team social worker (allocated to them at the time of admission) as an ally who would accept that they were normal, loving parents. Tension visibly mounted on the ward prior to the case conference. It was difficult for ward staff to accept that parents who seemed genuinely concerned about their child and had a manifestly warm and loving relationship with her could also have harmed that child. Tamsin was always delighted to see her mother who was understandably frightened; the father took time off work in order to be with his wife and babies. The nurses felt they had been put in an impossible position as they felt they were being required to spy on the parents and to judge them. They coped, for the most part, by trying to ignore them, which increased the parents' sense of isolation and injustice. Nothing emerged from the history given to the social worker to raise any doubt in her mind that the parents had any special difficulty in coping with their twins. However, the paediatrician informed the case conference that extreme force had been used to fracture Tamsin's leg and, in the absence of an acceptable explanation, it was decided that the twins could not go home. The parents were incensed and threatened to remove Tamara immediately (Tamsin was still on traction and therefore had to remain in hospital). The paediatrician and the social worker informed them that a Place of Safety Order would be sought if they tried to remove either child. Eventually, after much expression of anger and hostility towards the social services department (directed at both the hospital and the area team social worker) the father confessed that he could not stand Tamsin's crying. In a moment of rage and frustration, when his wife had left the room, he had sharply twisted the baby's leg and had heard the bone break. When Tamsin was well enough to be discharged from hospital the father moved out of the house. Both parents worked along with the area team social worker on their own relationship problems, while the father worked on his feelings of frustration with regard to parenting two small babies. Two years later he was back with his family and the twins were no longer on the Child Protection Register.

Case example: a sexually abused child Tracy was a little girl of 5 whose mother had always experienced difficulty parenting her. The situation had recently come to a head and the area team social worker decided to remove Tracy on a Place of Safety Order. Her parents had agreed to her being received into voluntary care and she was placed with a foster family. Two weeks later, when Tracy was being bathed by her foster mother, she told her about her father's sexual abuse of her. She was admitted to hospital the following day for investigation. As is frequently the case with the sexual abuse of small children, there were no physical findings and she was returned to her foster mother, since she was in no danger of further abuse. The paediatric social worker and a woman police officer then made several visits to the foster home to obtain an account from the child herself of what had happened. With the use of play material, with dolls, and with drawings the child was gradually able to give a very similar account to the one she had given to her foster mother. The magistrates agreed to a full Care Order and Tracy remained with the foster parents while receiving psychiatric treatment.

Sexual abuse is altogether more complex than physical abuse and does not necessarily require an admission to hospital. Unlike physical abuse, there may be no immediate urgency to remove the child, whose life is unlikely to be in danger. It is better to be sure of the facts than to act hastily with insufficient grounds which may lead to a child being returned to an abusing family.

Much of the work in child protection involves working closely with colleagues, both social workers in the area team and colleagues within the hospital. By its very nature child protection is stressful and time-consuming. Every social worker is aware of the implications if wrong judgements are made. If children are not adequately protected society blames those who are responsible for their protection. If children are removed from their families without apparent justification the social services department is the butt of public criticism. In many ways the social worker is in a no-win situation. It is therefore of vital importance to the paediatric social worker to have the support of managers (through supervision and consultation) and medical colleagues in the hospital (by joint interviewing and regular discussion), and to work closely with colleagues in the area team. There may well be differences of opinion, but each of the professionals concerned must be able to listen to all of the evidence, must not have any preconceived ideas about who may be to blame, and above all should not feel that they have to make a decision alone.

8.6 Accident/acute illness

Perhaps one of the most graphic examples of crisis theory and intervention is a sudden admission to a paediatric intensive care unit. Picture a normally functioning family, coping adequately with life, suddenly pitched into an emergency situation calling for extraordinary emotional stamina and the ability to function in the face of extreme stress. All the family's resilience and coping mechanisms are called into play and may well prove inadequate to the task. Crisis theory is seen to be immediately relevant and is the obvious theoretical framework for social work intervention. The theory of a period of temporary disequilibrium (caused by a stressful life event) when one's usual way of coping is either irrelevant, inappropriate or inadequate to the task was explored by Parad and others.[5] Intervention is based on helping the person to develop alternate or more adequate strategies such as support, practical advice and help, and partialising the tasks is at hand.

Case example: the crisis of a road traffic accident Mr and Mrs Andrews, a young professional couple, were returning home from a holiday weekend with their two children, Alexander aged 8 and David 6. They had had a late start on the return journey and Mr Andrews was in a hurry to get back as he had several important business matters to attend to. Everyone was tired and the children were quarrelling when Mr Andrews swerved to avoid on oncoming lorry and the car went out of control. Mr Andrews died at the scene of the accident and his wife lived for only a few hours in hospital. The children were admitted to the paediatric intensive care unit in a serious condition. The police finally located the nearest relative, an elderly aunt who lived eighty miles away, and she came during the night to be with the children. She was stressed, shocked, tired, and at times distraught.

The social worker was asked to see her the next day. The initial interviews primarily consisted of listening to her account of the accident and her feelings about it. In her state of shock (and at times denial) she kept repeating the description of the accident as told her by the police, in an attempt to accept it as a reality. On her own, now resident in the hospital, away from her friends and relatives she was thrown into a stressful situation of extreme intensity. The social worker focused on the immediate problems faced by her client at that stage. Together they considered ways of telling the children about the death of their parents. They discussed the need to register the deaths and make the funeral arrangements. Friends and employers had to be contacted to inform them of the accident. Arrangements had to be made for the aunt to be resident at the hospital and for her to cash her pension etc. Possible avenues of support for both the children and their aunt had to be identified, namely communicating with the family's friends and the childrens' school. The social worker contacted some of the aunt's friends and relatives, urging them to visit her and give her badly needed support. The family friends came to visit the children and were immensely helpful. Alexander and David, frightened and shocked in the hospital setting, confronted with an overwhelming loss, were comforted, not only by their aunt whom they knew well and with whom they had spent many holidays, but also by friends of their parents who talked to them gently about their mother and father and brought in family photographs.

The help of other professionals was enlisted in an attempt to support the family. A child psychiatrist was involved in a consultative capacity to help the ward staff, the ward teacher, and the family friends interact with the children in a more helpful way. A solicitor was contacted to handle the legal complexities and the children were made wards of court. Inter-professional meetings were established on the ward once a week in order to facilitate communication and to ensure that everyone worked closely as a team. This prevented conflicting advice being given and also ensured that all the professionals concerned received adequate support.

Bereavement counselling was undertaken with the aunt to help her verbalise her feelings of shock and disbelief. She was given the opportunity to cry and to express her anger as well as her feelings of bewilderment and pain. Thus the process of grieving was facilitated and she slowly began to assume more responsibility for practical details and to move from her own feelings of grief to try to meet the needs of the children.

The children, in effect, took a great deal longer to assimilate their loss, and it was not until several months after the accident that they began to show their feelings and talk about their parents. A memorial service was arranged two months later which the children and their aunt were encouraged to attend. Given the warm and loving support of extended family and friends they were at last able to reveal some of their distress. The child psychiatrist helped by interpreting their behaviour and emphasising that their reactions were normal under the circumstances.

Following discharge the children went to live with their aunt in another part of the country. The social worker remained concerned about their emotional well-being and took care to ensure that a psychiatrist would be available to them should they need ongoing help in the future. Contact was maintained with the aunt and referrals made to the local social services department and to a local solicitor who represented the aunt in the custody hearings.

Help given at salient points resulted in re-establishment of previous coping capacities, and hopefully an emotionally healthy start to the inevitably long and painful bereavement process.

Case example: the crisis of a serious surgical condition
Zara was transferred to the paediatric intensive care unit immediately after her birth became she was born with a serious congenital malformation of her oesophagus (trans-oesophagael fistula). This necessitates immediate surgery and sometimes results in months of being nursed on the intensive care unit on a ventilator (life-support machine) and being tube fed.

Zara's mother Kate was a single girl of 17 who lived with her supportive mother. However, Kate lived in a city thirty-five miles from the hospital and had no friends or relatives nearby. She was precipitated into the crisis of facing a situation for which she was totally unprepared, namely the birth of a baby with serious medical problems, coupled with the stress of adjusting to parenthood. While resident in the hospital Kate felt emotionally isolated and distressed without the support of her mother. She could not tolerate the idea of separation from the baby, feeling she had to remain in the hospital. Although she longed to comfort and hold her baby she felt impotent when confronted by the expert nursing staff on ITU and fearful of the complicated machinery. She was able only to hold the baby's hand and sit for hours by her cot as a passive onlooker. In relation to ward staff she was diffident and reluctant to ask many questions. Financial problems were also apparent and she needed immediate help in negotiating with the DSS.

The social worker was faced with a number of tasks. First, Kate needed help to work through her often confused feelings about the baby and her feelings of guilt at having caused the problem (as she believed). Secondly, the social worker was able to link up with Kate's mother and health visitor in order to ensure a supportive network when Kate eventually was able to go home. Immediate financial assistance was granted from the hospital Samaritan Fund and visiting costs were organised by applying to the DSS when Kate went home. Part of the social worker's role was to help interpret Kate's reactions to the ward staff and to help Kate understand the ward system and how it worked.

The work undertaken in cases such as those described falls into several distinct categories, as follows:

1. Advice on management of practical problems. It would seem to be important to offer practical help on a continuum. This involves initially adopting a strongly proactive role, taking over much of the decision-making from the client, who is thus freed to regress and grieve. Gradually the client can begin to tackle practical tasks independently until normal function is restored. Practical input at the beginning can focus on everything from the trivial (helping to make telephone calls, finding the hospital canteen, and arranging accommodation) to the more complex (liaising with solicitors and employers, making funeral arrangements, and organising the care of other children in the family).

2. Liaison with community networks. In a crisis situation the client needs a firm supportive network, not only from family and friends, but also from community services (e.g. clergy, area team social workers, psychiatric services). The hospital social worker can forge

and foster these links, maintaining contact with the outside agencies, interpreting the situation to them as it changes and trying to gear appropriate help at the right time. For example, contacting a client's employer, and perhaps arranging for paid sick leave, or asking the local social services department to make arrangements for the care of siblings can greatly ease the stress on the client.

3. Timing of intervention. Frequent brief contacts with a family in crisis are often more effective than lengthy single interviews. The client's concentration span is often adversely affected under stress and different aspects of the problem will only gradually emerge. If the social worker is able to tune-in frequently to the changes of emphasis and concern, the client feels supported and does not store up problems and difficulties, which can become overwhelming in their intensity.

4. Coping with feelings. In crisis situations the defences are lowered and therefore it is easier to talk about feelings. The social worker can help clients express the many conflicting feelings they may be experiencing, which is in itself therapeutic and helps to begin the difficult process of grief work. Care must be taken to ensure that communications are eased and fostered between close relatives involved. All too often a parent or child will find it difficult to express their feelings to those closest to them and it can be very helpful if they are enabled to do this with the help of an objective third party.

5. The social worker as patient's advocate. The social worker can usefully represent the client's feelings or wishes towards staff, thus avoiding misconceptions and communication problems. Often in a stressful situation parents are unable to take in medical information accurately. The social worker can explain to the staff involved that information may need to be repeated, often in increasing detail, as the parents move from initial reactions of shock to an ability to absorb and retain what they are being told.

We have thus seen how social work intervention in a paediatric intensive care unit is geared to the here and now, focusing on practical tasks as well as counselling services. Timing of intervention can also be important, with frequent brief sessions sensitively tuned to the needs of the patient and family.

8.7   Out-patients

A child and her family's contact with the hospital are sometimes focused on visits to an out-patient clinic where diagnosis and prospective management are explained at an out-patient's appointment. This contact may continue over a period of many years, for example in the management of a chronic condition such as one of the epilepsies.

The prolonged period between first parental concerns, through testing, to the diagnostic conclusion can be termed a 'crisis', although it may last some months. Social work intervention is often appropriate as crisis theory still applies.

Case example: a child with a deteriorating condition Brian first came to the notice of the hospital when he was 4 years old. He was developmentally delayed and was referred to a consultant paediatric neurologist because of his poor speech and immature behaviour. Her immediate suspicion was of a metabolic disease. The consultant felt that early social work contact would be important and with parental agreement the social worker joined in on consultations. David and Susan, the parents, were at first unaware of the doctor's fears, as yet unsubstantiated. However the social worker became a familiar figure over the lengthy period while physical and psychological testing was carried out.

This early 'latching on' time before it is certain if there is a major medical problem can be uncomfortable for the social worker before her role is clear to either party! However there is usually room for the sometimes maligned supportive contact. This may subsequently be remembered as an aspect of the caring face of the hospital by the relieved parent or can be the solid foundation for a useful relationship if things do not turn out so well.

Sadly in Brian's case a firm diagnosis was made of a very severe metabolic condition, caused by a recessive gene, which would result in Brian gradually losing the faculties he already had. There is no treatment to change the prognosis; only palliative management of symptoms. Tragically it was soon discovered that David and Susan's only other child had the same condition.

When the crucial test results were all back, arrangements were made by the social worker for meetings variously involving parents, grandparents, health visitor, consultant and social worker. This allowed parents time to discuss the final diagnosis and as much of the outlook as they wished. David and Susan were given the opportunity to be alone after the initial consultation to compose themselves for the outside world. The social worker's involvement of grandparents acknowledged their crucial role in a close network of family and friends. It was clearly difficult to accept and understand such a devastating diagnosis. The attitude and understanding of those close to such families is as significant in affecting how families subsequently cope as any professional input. This facilitating role had the advantage of increasing the social worker's knowledge of a rare condition. This is important if the family are to have confidence in the social worker. It allows her to plan possible future needs for resources, and for the family she may be the only non-medical person who can understand without their having to go into lengthy and painful explanations.

It is important to be sensitive to the needs of individual families. Some parents are offended by the mention of the management of practical details when they are still in the raw early stages of grieving. Others give immediate thought to 'How will I cope?' and need reassurance about available resources.

The social worker made early mention of the appropriate association run by and for parents of similarly affected children which offers mutual support and information. David and Susan made contact when the time seemed right for them and found the association valuable.

There are a number of financial benefits available to

parents with chronically sick or disabled children. Attendance Allowance is payable where a child over 2 years of age has needed either frequent supervision to avoid danger or attention in connection with bodily functions for more than six months. This must be greater than the attention needed by a healthy child of the same age. Invalid Care Allowance can be claimed by someone caring for the child in receipt of Attendance Allowance, if the carer is not in gainful employment or in receipt of certain other benefits. Mobility Allowance is payable where a child over the age of 5 is virtually or totally unable to walk or where the exertion would be a risk to health.

Two government financed agencies can be approached by families with severely disabled children. The Independent Living Fund assists where families are on a very low income and need to pay someone to help look after their affected child. The Family Fund will help with some major items needed to relieve families (on or below moderate income) such as a washing machine, a fridge-freezer, or a family holiday.[6,7]

In this case Attendance Allowance, Invalid Care Allowance and Mobility Allowance were successfully obtained, eventually! When an appeal was necessary the social worker's close contacts in the hospital were crucial. Family Fund helped with a new washing machine and a scrubbable carpet for incontinent children who would never now be toilet trained.

Early arrangements were made by the consultant for a detailed developmental assessment of Brian at the local multi professional assessment centre for handicapped children. Four day-visits allowed consideration of all aspects of the child by resident and visiting specialists and a thorough check of provision was made to ensure that the family was enabled to care for the child with the least stress to them and greatest gain to the child. This intensive week involved the social worker closely. She made a prior home visit in order to explain the workings of the unit to parents and to establish in detail the parents' anxieties and hopes relating to the assessment. A report was made to the staff at the centre as an introduction to the family and their needs. The social worker subsequently ensured that David and Susan felt that their concerns had been addressed and she also dealt with matters arising with implications for social work service.

In the early months the extended family were able to offer sufficient relief by babysitting and having the children to stay overnight. After about a year respite care at a residential unit was accepted and later a children's hospice offered help allowing David and Susan more flexibility in placing both children.

The social worker kept in touch by making occasional home visits and joining out-patient consultations. Sadly the children deteriorated noticeably losing most speech and concentration. Susan, after the initial trauma, has coped well. She loves her children and manages them with great skill and understanding. She is able to separate from them to get the breaks she and her husband need while missing them while they are away. Both parents suffer the chronic sorrow described by Olshanky[8] and Nolan[9] but the structure of support accepted was sufficient to keep the family functioning.

Initial intensive input by the social worker, amongst others, was highly productive in helping the whole family settle to the task of caring for two children with a limited life expectancy and increasing dependency. As a hospital-based worker she was in a position to liaise closely with colleagues in the hospitals and with outside agencies, both statutory and voluntary.

8.8   Information giving and counselling

Case examples: Three girls with epilepsy

1. Samantha first had recognised seizures at 5 years which caused terrific fears in her family. They were angry and distressed and initially disbelieving of the diagnosis in their 'perfect' only child. They had first to lay aside their own prejudices against those with epilepsy. They mistakenly believed the seizures to have been caused by an unrelated infection and blamed their GP for not tackling the latter more aggressively. In

common with many parents, when they first witnessed Samantha having a major seizure they thought that their child was going to die.

The first medication tried had no effect thus confirming the frantic parents' distrust of the medical profession. A scan showed minor abnormalities of the brain structure and psychological testing was suggested to see if there were any specific cognitive problems. This plan enraged a distressed mother already burdened with guilty, as yet unexpressed, fears that family problems had caused the condition. The number of seizures was dramatically reduced with the next drug tried. However, grandparents still treated her as a 'sick' child.

Early social work counselling was successful in modifying family attitudes to Samantha's epilepsy. The social worker supplied Epilepsy Association literature appropriate to Samantha's age and type of epilepsy. Her parents had the time to express their fears allowing the social worker to reassure them that many families experienced similar feelings. They were encouraged to talk in simple terms to Samantha about her condition when they felt she was ready and they were given a simple book for children, a good basis for parent-child discussion.

Samantha's epilepsy subsequently went through unsettled and worrying phases but she coped cheerfully with necessary restrictions, such as wearing a helmet, whereas she had initially exhibited demanding and difficult behaviour overall.

Pond and Bidwell drew attention to the significance of parental attitudes evoked by epilepsy, especially at a very early stage, in determining the child's later adjustment.[10] When Ward and Bower studied epileptic children and their families visiting out-patients, they found that a number interviewed expressed the wish that they could have had the chance to talk to a social worker at a much earlier stage.[11] Many consciously used the opportunity thus provided to talk out some of their difficulties and expressed their appreciation of it. The study also pointed out that the out-patient clinic does not always provide an atmosphere likely to encourage confidences especially when restless children are around. Home visits from the hospital base are indeed an integral part of work with such families. They may be more relaxed and less intimidated when talking on home territory. Children and adults alike feel more in control. Hospitality can be offered in exchange for help. The relationship between social worker and client is more egalitarian and thus more comfortable, at least for the family!

2. Lizzie, in contrast to Samantha, had never had any explanation or mention of the fact that she had epilepsy; it was a family secret. When the social worker met her, four years after diagnosis, she felt this explained Lizzie's lack of confidence and particular vulnerability to teasing at school. With parental agreement, she was given some literature. Interestingly, it was her older sister who first read the book. She had been very concerned about her sister having witnessed, but not understood, her seizures. The effect on siblings of a child with a chronic condition can be significant but easily ignored when the focus is on the sick child.

3. When she first met the social worker Joanna was 12 and had suffered from epilepsy for some years, as had a close relative. Although generally a well-adjusted child she was experiencing frequent absence attacks (minor epilepsy) which affected her concentration, provoked teasing at school and drastically interfered with learning at a time of transfer to secondary school. She was miserable at being so 'stupid' that she couldn't even ride a bike. The first interview at her home was difficult as she was feeling shy and having noticeable absence attacks. However her mother later reported that she had taken in a great deal more than it had appeared. One book's representation appealed to her as it showed everyone to have some handicap either obvious or hidden; from obesity or wearing glasses to epilepsy. She took a more outgoing stance about her epilepsy and with additional special help

with schoolwork conquered her feelings of being less worthwhile than other people. In a few subsequent sessions over several years she talked with the social worker about her feelings about the necessary restrictions on her, and was better able to appreciate the balance between safety and independence already thought through by her mother. A single outing arranged with other children with troubling epilepsy in normal school did much to emphasise her new knowledge that she was not alone and increased her self respect.

Such children's conditions are not necessarily severe in medical terms, but within the context of each individual family are of great significance. Preventive social work intervention, near the time of diagnosis, is particularly time effective and promotes a healthy adjustment to a disease or condition which may intrinsically interfere with the pattern of normal life. It ensures that child and family minimalise the deleterious effect. It encourages the child to grow up both confident and comfortable in herself.

Paediatric social work deals with children and their families at times of particular vulnerability. Intervention is successful in situations varying between dramatic life-threatening circumstances and longer periods of stress and strain where need is less obvious. Based in hospital, as part of a multidisciplinary team, social work help is available at the point of need and in a context acceptable to most families. A good service responds quickly at a time of crisis but also offers lower key, long-term assistance.

Notes

1. A life-threatening illness involving serious problems of the lungs and digestive system. The victim usually survives to early adult life but can die in childhood if severely affected.
2. Murray Parkes, Colin, *Studies of Grief in Adult Life*, Harmondsworth: Penguin, 1980.
3. Parton, N., *The Politics of Child Abuse*, London: Macmillan, 1985.
4. Douglas, Anthony, 'All you need to know to enjoy case conferences', *Social Work Today*, 16 March 1989.
5. Parad, H. J. (ed.), *Crisis Intervention: Selected readings*, Family Services Association of America, 1978.

6. DSS leaflets: FB 2, NI 243, NI 212, NI 205.
7. Fact sheet, *Child Disability Benefits and Other Forms of Help*, Contact A Family, 16 Strutton Ground, London SW1P 2HP, September 1988.
8. Olshanky, Simon, 'Chronic sorrow: a response to having a mentally defective child', *Social Casework*, **43**, 1962, pp. 190–3.
9. Nolan, R., *Counselling Parents of the Mentally Retarded*, Springfields, Illinois: C. C. Thomas, 1970.
10. Pond, D. A., and Bidwell, B. H., *A Survey of Epilepsy in Fourteen General Practices*, *Epilepsia*, **1**, 1960.
11. Ward, F., and Bower, B. D., 'A study of certain social aspects of epilepsy in childhood, *Developmental Medicine and Child Neurology, Supplement 39*, **20**, 1.

Suggestions for further reading

Bancroft, J., 'Crisis intervention', in: *An Introduction to the Psychotherapies*, Oxford: OUP, 1979.

Beran, R., *Learning about Epilepsy*, Medican Education Services, 1982.

Burton, L., *The Care of the Child facing Death*, London: Routledge & Kegan Paul, 1974.

DHSS and The Welsh Office, *Working together: A guide to arrangements for inter-agency co-operation for the protection of children*, London: HMSO, 1983.

Gilbert, P., *Mental Handicap: A practical guide for social workers*, London: Community Care Publications, 1986.

Jones, D., *Interviewing the Sexually Abused Child*, London: Royal Society of Medicine, 1988.

Lansdown, R., The development of the concept of death and its relationship to communication with dying children, in: *Current Issues in Clinical Psychology*, E. Karas (ed.), London: Plenum, 1987.

Sarnoff Schieff H., *The Bereaved Parent*, London: Souvenir, 1977.

CHAPTER 9

The elderly person as patient and client

MARGARET COPPEARD

9.1　The ageing process

Ageing is a natural process. Ageism or age discrimination is a condition imposed by society and the dictates of the economy.[1] Any person who has reached pensionable age may well be labelled 'geriatric', 'elderly' or 'pensioner'. But what does this mean? At a certain age society begins to make assumptions based on various stereotypes. An older couple are seen as having the freedom to enjoy themselves with time and money to do what they want. They have access to free bus passes, cheap holidays out of season and other concessions. Alternatively, the 'pensioner' is seen as a poor person living alone, subject to hypothermia in winter and needing charity from those who are productive members of society. Other stereotypes are of aimless bumbling to which the media contributes in various situation comedies where the elderly characters are shown as interfering busybodies having nothing useful to fill their days. The negative image is reinforced in sketches of the old man with watery eyes and slipping teeth and in a number of such programmes where confused old people are used as figures of fun. Why is this necessary? Is it to protect and defend younger people from the uncomfortable fact of their loss of youth?

The reality for the individual or couple who have reached pensionable age is that they may well have suffered loss of status, friends, finance and aims because of retirement but do not feel either elderly or geriatric. However, they are no longer seen to be economically productive and have become members of an identified group purely on the basis of reaching a certain age. (Teenage is the only comparable situation!)

Attitudes may well be changing and, in the situation which

may obtain in a few years when there will be more elderly people than wage-earners it is being suggested that the elderly will become a valued economic resource and the age of retirement will go up. Will this mean that terms like 'elderly' and 'geriatric' will disappear? Certainly many newly retired people hold well-paid part-time jobs, do very useful voluntary work and are in the majority as unpaid carers of the frail elderly. Most elderly people will continue for many years past retirement without any recourse to social work intervention and only accident or illness may change circumstances and ability to manage and so necessitate help from statutory services.

To the elderly person old age is generally at least five years on even if she is 90! The ageing process begins at birth and as we get older the losses accumulate until, through trauma or illness, loss of health and approaching death have to be acknowledged. Proust says: 'Adolescents who last long enough are what life makes old men out of' and it is this concept, that everyone has a present and future, that the person in the hospital bed is an individual who has family and friends, hopes and fears, wishes, likes and dislikes, that social workers working with the elderly person in hospital must hold to.

The elderly are probably the largest group of people who will be referred to the hospital social worker. In one district general hospital 70 per cent of referrals for one year were for people over pensionable age and most of these were for people of 80 and over although there were only 50 beds out of 350 that were designated 'acute elderly'.

The stay in hospital may be precipitated by increased frailty and falls, by an accident or the onset of an acute illness, and the way in which an elderly person is admitted to hospital is often traumatic. The admission, if not planned through a domiciliary visit from the consultant for the elderly or resulting from an out-patient appointment, will be through the accident and emergency department at the local hospital and at this point the patient may be unable to stand or walk, may be disorientated and frightened and will be feeling ill and uncomfortable and probably in pain.

Case example: To any social worker who has worked in a hospital and covered duty in the accident and emergency department the story of Mrs Smith and her admission to hospital will be familiar.

Mrs Smith had fallen as she went out to the lavatory in the middle of the night. She could not get up off the floor and was found by her home help when she came in next morning. Mrs Smith was cold, hungry and frightened. The home help called an ambulance and Mrs Smith was taken to the local hospital accident and emergency department. She was examined by a doctor, had X-rays and blood tests and was found to have broken her wrist but there was no reason to admit her to a hospital ward and a social worker was called to arrange for services so that she could go home. Mrs Smith explained that her daughter was on holiday abroad and her son lived about fifty miles away; although he always rang at lunchtime she didn't see him much and didn't get on with his wife. She had a home help once a week to do the housework and she didn't like to bother the neighbours who were at work all day. The social worker asked her to sit up and to get off the bed to see how far she could walk but she couldn't Mrs Smith was by now exhausted and feeling very alone. She told the social worker that she was frightened to go home and just wanted to stay somewhere safe until her daughter came back from holiday. The social worker had to negotiate on Mrs Smith's behalf to try to get her into a hospital bed or into a residential home although Mrs Smith's degree of dependency at that point may well have precluded the latter option since she was unable to use her walking frame. Mrs Smith was admitted to a hospital ward but the length of time, the protracted discussion and the uncertainty of the outcome did nothing to help her and may well have left her feeling she was taking a bed inappropriately.

The social worker needed skills of assessment and advocacy, and insight into the patient's needs and wishes to achieve a satisfactory solution. This is particularly pertinent at a time when resources are scarce and many consultants are very concerned not to admit for what are considered to be social reasons.

9.2 The social worker as advocate and educator

In considering social work with the elderly person the role of
the social worker in the hospital as advocate for the patient is
probably the most positive and important. Above every other
consideration must come the right of the elderly person to choose
where to live, how to live and where to die. It is up to the social
worker to empower that person to give her the courage or to
support her in whatever decision she wishes to take even if it is
contrary to the advice of the doctors or the wishes of her family.
For an old lady who may be confined to one room, prone to falls,
having meals on wheels seven days a week and the home help
twice a day it may seem to the outside observer that the obvious
solution is for her to go into the comfort and safety of an elderly
persons' home. However, if she chooses, despite all advice to the
contrary, to stay in her one room that is her right. It is her link
with the past, with her memories, it is familiar, it is her home.

The legal framework beginning with the National Assistance
Act 1948, Section 47(1), makes it quite clear that the following
criteria are necessary before compulsory action to remove an
elderly person from the home is taken:

(a) [the elderly persons] are suffering from grave chronic disease or,
being aged infirm or physically incapacitated, are living in insanitary
conditions and

(b) are unable to devote to themselves and are not receiving from
other persons proper care and attention.[2]

The only other criterion is that the person is suffering from a
mental illness and is sectionable under the Mental Health Act
1983.

The social worker may well come into conflict with every other
discipline within the hospital and with families or neighbours if
she supports the elderly person in her insistence in staying at
home. With frail elderly people being cared for more frequently
in the community the social worker will inevitably be drawn into
the debate about risk-taking. Whose risk? What is an acceptable
risk? If one accepts that a person may drive a car or fly round
the world with all the associated dangers or an explorer may
walk to the South Pole, a mountain climber may scale the most
dangerous peaks, a motor-cyclist may ride in the Manx T T races

— all with a high risk of fatality — why does it cause so much heart searching and concern when a frail elderly person expresses the wish to return home and run the risk of falling again and is there any difference? Have we as a society the right to impose custodial care in the name of caring on people because their health is failing? In these situations the social worker will often walk a tightrope.

> *Case example*: Ada was in her late 80s and had a large family. They, together with her GP and the consultant geriatrician at the local hospital, all insisted that she should go into residential care but Ada, who was very deaf and a determined, rather eccentric and very frail lady, wanted to stay in her own home. She eventually and reluctantly accepted support from social services and, although her family refused to visit her because she wouldn't go into residential care, took no part in supporting her and to the end of her life rarely visited her, she was where she wanted to be and only went into hospital for the last few days of her life. She confided to the social worker: 'You see, I am so lonely when I am with people because I can't hear them!'.

Multi-disciplinary working, the team made up of nurses, doctors, social workers, physiotherapists and occupational therapists, can be a positive forum for discussing different points of view and since the social worker is the link with community services she may need to spend much time discussing services and options with her colleagues in this team in order to gain their confidence for what may well be considered to be a risky discharge.

For many people the doctor is a figure of authority and this combined with the often paternalistic effect of the institution can give a hospital patient the idea that she has no right to decide about her future, that everything is in the hands of someone else. She may be told she can no longer cope at home and should go into residential care. She may be told that she is to be made into a long-stay patient because she cannot manage. In these cases the social worker's role is to discover the patient's wishes and to give her the opportunity to explore all the options.

Case example: The social worker realised that Mr A. who was in his 90s and waiting to be transferred to a long-stay bed, wanted to go home but, because of his frailty and age, rehabilitation had not been considered. The social worker, whilst recognising that Mr A. might well be unrealistic, respected his wishes and persuaded the occupational therapist to do a home visit. As a result of the home visit Mr A. was able to say that he would not be able to manage and that he wished to sell his home and enter a private nursing home. This he did and settled very happily. He made his own choice, he was still in control of his life, the social worker had empowered him to make his own decision.

A social worker acting as the patient's advocate may have to negotiate with the DSS for all benefits available, perhaps with the Independent Living Fund, with charities and with the local authority for services. This last can be frustrating and time consuming because very rarely does the social worker in hospital actually hold the key to unlock the resource and can only recommend. When a scarce resource like a day centre placement is suggested as an essential part of the discharge package, a long wait while residential services assess the request and decide on the appropriateness of the placement can be frustrating for the social worker and client alike and a successful outcome may depend on the patience of the consultant who may well find it difficult to understand why the hospital social worker's recommendation is not enough. Informal networks with colleagues in the community and recognition of the complementarity of each other's role is vital if successful discharges are to be achieved in difficult situations. Some authorities have put a home care organiser with a team of home care workers into the hospital. They work closely with the social work team and hospital personnel and will undertake intensive rehabilitation work for a short period before transferring the case to their area colleagues once the client is settled at home. As elderly patients are now discharged much more quickly and therefore may be more vulnerable, hospital social workers could be in a position to recommend similar initiatives to their local authorities in order to prevent immediate re-admissions and the 'revolving door' syndrome.

Perhaps the most difficult area of advocacy is with the families of the elderly person. The social worker can recognise the stress under which they have been, the constant fear and worry and for a short while this has been lifted. Much work may be needed to convince the family of the elderly person's rights to return home. The social worker must take care not to collude with relatives because they have communicated their anxiety and distress at the idea of discharge. Alternatively, the social worker must not be intimidated by the family who become aggressive and try to blackmail the social worker with threats about her responsibility if the patient falls or is not safe at home.

The problem is that it is much easier for an elderly person to become a hospital patient than to cease to be one. There are a number of reasons for this. The 'social space' in which the person has been living may close behind him on admission so that he cannot get back. A family may heave a sigh of relief having realised, perhaps for the first time, what a burden it has been carrying and say 'He's not coming back here!' A landlord may take the opportunity to re-possess his house or the warden of a sheltered housing complex say 'He needs too much nursing now, I can't cope!'. Ironically, it is often the person who would appear to be most at risk, who lives alone in his own home, who is in least danger of having his social space close up on him.[3]

9.3   Working with carers

If care in the community is to work then attention must be paid to the needs of the carers who may often themselves be retired. It is vital to get the patient's permission to begin to build up a picture of the elderly person's networks and to make contact with closest relatives and carers as soon as possible after the admission to the hospital ward. Experience shows that however isolated and neglected the patient appears it is rare indeed that there is not some relative with whom she has some sort of contact. One such example was an elderly lady who gave small and tantalising details about her past. When she died the Official Solicitor was unable to trace from her belongings any member of her family or any friend and her next of kin was given as her ex-landlady of only seven years although it was known that she had been one of three sisters who were soubrettes in the 1920s!

Who is the carer and why has that person assumed the role? Very frequently it is a daughter who, it is taken for granted, will devote herself to her aged parent. Mrs B. was brought to accident and emergency by her daughter and son-in-law. She was 100 and they were in their late 70s. They had been on holiday and Mrs B. had been in the local elderly persons' home which she already knew from previous visits. Mrs B.'s health had deteriorated rapidly during the two weeks and it was felt she was pining as tests had revealed no illness. Mrs B. lived alone in the house she had moved to as a bride. Her daughter and son-in-law lived about five minutes walk away. One or other went first thing every morning to get her up then they took lunch and cooked it in her kitchen for them all. There was another visit in the evening to help her get to bed. They had never asked for help from anyone but now felt that with mother ill and frail they could no longer cope. They were anxious, frightened and already tired. We discussed options and with the help of the local home care organiser arranged a night sitter for that night, a home help to go in first thing every morning at least for the next week and the assurance that there were people to share the burden. Furthermore they were able to talk about their fear that Mrs B. would die alone or fall and that people would blame them because she had been left!

Sometimes it is the spouse, an unmarried son or a long-standing friend who devotedly nurses the ailing partner to the detriment of his own health. Mrs C. was a very large and demanding lady heavily handicapped with rheumatoid arthritis. Mr C. was a large dour ex-docker. His leg ulcers were getting increasingly painful but she would never accept his needs and he never complained, just looked after her and obeyed every demand. He eventually had to go into hospital and because she could do nothing for herself she had to go into the local geriatric long-stay ward. She was very angry with him and felt he was making a fuss about nothing and when he died and she had to go into a nursing home her anger knew no bounds. She never at any time expressed any concern about his pain or regret at his death. An extreme case? Yes, but why did he allow himself to get into such a situation? One can speculate; perhaps guilt that he was able and she was so handicapped; perhaps she had always been the dominant partner and the behaviour pattern of demand and obey could not be altered; perhaps a very deep sense of duty; perhaps a need to care; perhaps a deep love. There were elements of all these but he could not talk about his feelings nor acknowledge them. Likewise for her there was a very real need for self-preservation but she had no insight into his needs or her own character.

Whatever the relationship, it should not be taken for granted that that person can or is willing to spend twenty-four hours in the company of the frail person. It is essential for the social worker to recognise the family dynamics in these situations. Is the carer guilt-ridden for any reason? Has the role reversal of child now parent been acknowledged and accepted? Is the carer over-protective and the elderly person unable to achieve some sort of normality in living? It is the task of the social worker to help the carer by devising help from various agencies individually tailored for clients and carers. This is often called care packaging and will entail a careful assessment of the needs and routines of the client and without this support the carer may quickly collapse and the elderly person return to hospital.

A very difficult situation can occur when the family won't allow any help, feeling that they should bear the burden and it is when the carer finally cracks that social services are called in. Within hospital social work, this can be on the admission of the elderly person to hospital. It may be at this point that the social worker can help the carers to acknowledge their anger and its many facets. Anger because the rest of the family are refusing to take a share in the caring role, anger at being tied down and the guilt because of the anger. There is pain at the loss of a loved parent who has to be looked after like a child and this can be particularly difficult when the elderly person has become demented. It can also be at this point that the family reject the elderly relative and the social worker needs to be very aware of this possibility and the reasons if she is to help the patient, her client, to achieve any sort of independence on discharge.

A scenario familiar to the social worker in hospital is to be asked to tell the old person she can't return home or to be asked to get her into a residential home 'just for a short holiday', the family having every intention of leaving her there. Such requests should be firmly refused by the social worker remembering the right of the elderly person to choose and also the fact that the client simply won't believe the social worker. Honesty and openness must always be encouraged and it may take many hours of counselling before the family are able to appreciate the elderly person's point of view. The process may involve dealing with the relatives' anger and anxiety during which the elderly person can be left isolated and very bewildered.

Case example: Mrs Brown lived next door to her daughter Ethel who popped in two or three times a day and cooked all her meals. Ethel had not been on holiday for some years because she could not leave her mother, but now her husband Fred had retired and the children had moved up north they needed some free time. Ethel's brother and his wife who also lived near them could not commit themselves to help with mother as neither had very good health and were very busy in the golf club. Mrs Brown was admitted to hospital and at first Ethel visited regularly. As her mother's health improved and discharge was being planned the doctors and social worker saw Ethel and discussed what help was available. Ethel had never had any help and at first said she didn't need any, then as the date of discharge came nearer she said she couldn't manage her mother any longer. The social worker again suggested possible help that might be available but Ethel insisted that her mother needed twenty-four hour supervision and that she couldn't give it. She said her mother would be at risk. Fred became involved and there was a very heated discussion when Fred shouted at the social worker. There were also angry telephone calls from Ethel and Fred's children demanding help for the grandmother. Ethel's visits became irregular, the social worker left messages to ask Ethel to contact her, then she tried to be on the ward at Ethel's visiting times but somehow Ethel was never there and the telephone was never answered and then a message came that Ethel was unwell. Mrs Brown became very upset and anxious about going home. She missed her daughter's visits and her health began to deteriorate. She wanted to get out of hospital and to go and live with Ethel. The nursing staff became involved, telling Mrs Brown that she wouldn't manage at home alone and that she needed to be cared for in 'a nice place'. Mrs Brown appeared to agree but when the social worker talked to her about residential accommodation she said her daughter would decide for her. All was at stalemate, no home visit could be arranged as Ethel held the key to Mrs Brown's house and refused to release it. Eventually the social worker managed to meet Fred and although initially things looked very black both he and Ethel were able to discuss the whole situation, acknowledge their frustration, fears and anger and the control they were trying to take over Mrs Brown's life. Because they were enabled to talk more deeply about their feelings Mrs Brown was able to tell about her own loneliness in her home and her need for company and, although she returned home and went to a day centre for a while, she eventually decided to go into a residential home.

When an elderly spouse rejects their partner the social worker is presented with a difficult dilemma. Both may be elderly and perhaps it is a sense of self-preservation that has brought about this action because of heavy nursing needs but it may be that the social worker is being asked to contrive a decent and acceptable separation because for years the couple have hated each other. In either of these situations the social worker must discover what are the wishes of the patient. It may call for a great deal of ingenuity to help that person return home but it is one partner's home as much as it is the other's and he or she has every right to return.

Case example: Mr H., in his late 70s, suffered a stroke and although he regained some mobility he needed help into and out of bed and to the lavatory and washing. His speech and understanding were somewhat impaired. Mrs H. insisted she could not have her husband home, that the nursing demands were too heavy for her and that he should stay in hospital or go into an elderly person's home. Mr H., as far as it was possible to establish, longed to get back to his home, his garden and his wife's cooking. After several interviews with Mrs H. it became clear that the marriage had ended long ago. Mrs H., an active lady, had her own interests outside the home and went on holidays abroad with a group of friends while Mr H. was perfectly happy to watch television and tend his garden. The illusion of a marriage was preserved because she had pride in cooking and keeping house but they had slept in different rooms for many years and barely communicated. Now, the idea that she would have physical and intimate contact with this man whom she loathed was too much for her and she was seizing the opportunity to end the relationship. The solution was to treat Mr H. as a lodger in the household. Mrs H. was prepared to cook and clean and the social worker coordinated the necessary nursing, domiciliary and day-care services.

An area which has to be considered and carefully and sensitively handled by the social worker is the abuse of the elderly by a carer. The perpetrator will feel ashamed and afraid and the elderly person is generally very protective and will not admit how the bruise or fall occurred but it is worth being very watchful if an elderly person for no apparent reason appears afraid to go home from hospital. An old lady living with a very caring son began to try to prolong her stay in hospital and then to talk about her son's embarrassment at cleaning her 'private parts', although there was no obvious reason for him to have to do so. On meeting the son it became evident that his behaviour was rigid and regimented to the point of abnormality. Eventually a grand-daughter spoke to the social worker and explained that the whole family were afraid of him and that once home no other member of the family would be allowed to visit or see the old lady. The social worker suggested to her that she could go into an elderly persons' home if she was worried about her son's embarrassment (not a normal practice for the team!) and the look of relief that flooded her face and her subsequent recovery and happiness tended to confirm the original suspicions although the old lady never accused her son.

It has become one of the functions of the social worker in hospital to coordinate discharges for elderly persons, particularly if they are frail, to discuss the carer's role and to bring in other agencies, volunteers, and social services to assist in the task of caring. However, a carer who has shouldered the burden perhaps for several years may find it difficult to believe there is help and it may be necessary to bring together involved professionals and agencies and the relatives and the elderly person in an informal meeting. The group invited could include some or all of the following: a hospital and an area social worker, home care organiser, community occuptional therapist, district nurse, Cross Roads organiser, GP, consultant, ward nurse, patient, relative, hospital occupational therapist, physiotherapist and local voluntary groups. Such a group may be threatening for the patient and family but, sensitively handled by the chairperson and with the common aim to help the patient get home and the carer to continue to manage, it can be a positive exercise. An alternative, or possibly in addition, can be the home visit, a day-long visit when the elderly person has time to settle down, to look at her home again and when the various disciplines can visit individually and not all together. The carer can be given some idea of what it will be like when the elderly person returns and what is needed to manage, and services can be planned and integrated. To adopt such a strategy can be reassuring for the carer who has never asked for help particularly if the carer herself is frail. It also gives the client the opportunity to reflect on the reality of home, especially if she has been in hospital for some time and the admission was very traumatic. It can give the space to admit that she will not manage, is frightened of the loneliness and wants to make alternative arrangements, or even to come to terms with the need to move furniture around. Most of all it gives the opportunity to face the reality of what may be a very changed lifestyle to that which was enjoyed prior to entering hospital.

9.4   Residential care

Assessing the need for residential care and explaining the options and financial anomalies can create a difficult and demanding task for the social worker.

Local authorities were charged in Part 3 of the 1948 Act to provide 'residential accommodation for persons who by reason of age, infirmity or any other circumstances are in need of care and attention which is not otherwise available to them'. In a letter dated March 1988 addressed to Sally Greengross, Director of Age

Concern, Nicholas Scott, Minister of State for Social Security and the Disabled, wrote:

Decisions about the discharge of people from hospital are for the consultant in charge of the patient's care to make and must be made on clinical grounds. Financial considerations should not enter into the decision. Where it is decided that a patient requires continuing in-patient medical or nursing care, it falls to the NHS to supply it at no cost to the patient. The on-going care can be provided either by the patient remaining in an NHS hospital bed or for example by transfer to a private nursing home under contractual arrangements, with the NHS meeting the full cost and retaining the ultimate responsibility for the patient's care.[4]

Both these statements are open to many and varied interpretations and it does not appear that either has been tested in a court of law. It can, therefore, be the responsibility of the individual social worker to assess and advise on the appropriate establishment for the elderly person who does not wish to return home. There are no clear guidelines from either authority as to criteria of need for placement in one or other establishment although it is probable that there are many people in long-stay geriatric beds who are accepted by the consultant as needing that care but who would be more appropriately placed in residential care and similarly people in residential care who are very highly dependent and needing nursing care. Equally difficult is the determination of the patient's rights. Does the person wishing to go into residential care have the right to insist that it should be a local authority home? Does the patient needing nursing care have the right to insist on staying in an NHS hospital and what does 'in-patient nursing care' mean?

In theory there are five options.

1. *Local authority elderly persons' home*
   This is means-tested, there is often a long waiting list and people are admitted by need not position on the list. The intending resident must have a certain degree of mobility and independence.
2. *Private or voluntary residential care*
   If the applicant has no capital the DSS will contribute to a certain limit but since many homes are above this limit families or charities will be asked to top up. The person with

capital has no certainty that when her money is exhausted she will be able to stay in the home and it is this uncertainty that may cause a patient or family to decide against private care. Again the owner or officer-in-charge will expect a certain degree of independence.

3. *NHS nursing home*
   Very few of these have been established and for most hospital social workers and their clients this is not an option.

4. *Private nursing home*
   As with the residential homes but the cost may be even more prohibitive.

5. *Long-stay care in an NHS hospital*
   This is a resource which seems to be disappearing fast with the closure of long-stay geriatric wards in many hospitals and the emphasis on acute short admission to hospital and fast turnover.

An added complication for any social worker advising about residential care is the anomaly of cost. If a person is accepted as a long-stay patient in an NHS hospital there is a loss of state pension but, unlike admission to residential care or any form of private care, she may never have to make the decision to give up her home since no payment is incurred. It may well be that many of these problems will be resolved when the government guidelines are published with the new Act in 1991.

Who makes the decision that an elderly person in hospital should go into residential accommodation? Sadly, although theoretically it is the old person's decision and should be a positive option to living in the community, it may well have been suggested to her that she can no longer manage at home and she may feel she has to agree. Unfortunately if she refuses she may be seen as unrealistic and if she is re-admitted to hospital hands are raised in horror, everyone saying 'I told you so!', and the social worker who assisted the patient to return home is told: 'This can't go on!'. However, to give up one's home may well be the last loss before loss of life itself. It may be the last hope and link with the past and former identity. These feelings must be respected and the hospital social worker will need to spend time counselling about the reality of communal living and to give the patient the space and time to say goodbye to her home.

On the other hand, there are some elderly people who seem quite capable but, for various reasons, have lost the motivation or wish to return home. It may be loneliness or fear; it may be that the person has had a positive experience of communal living or has friends in elderly persons' home. For whatever reason, this person's wishes must be respected. The social worker will need to discuss the options available and to make sure the person is aware of the realities of the decision. Within many local authorities it is now likely that a request for residential care from a relatively active person would not be considered and the person may have no alternative to private care. The following interesting situation appeared to have no resolution. Mrs D. lived alone in a bungalow. She had no capital. She was an anxious and frail lady and her family were caring and concerned. Neither she nor her family would agree that she could manage at home although social services stated they could provide the necessary level of domiciliary care to maintain her in the community. She and her family refused to consider private care insisting that she had a right to expect local authority care. The authority had a long waiting list and, because they considered she could manage at home, Mrs D. was not a priority. The consultant then had to decide whether to insist on discharging Mrs D. back into the community and to face the consequences of his action.

The social worker can come under great pressure from the consultant to 'get the person out' and from family to 'do something' to find a place. The social worker in turn may well feel angry and impotent because she does not hold the key to unlock the resource. Whilst the aim of both hospital staff and hospital social workers is to return a patient to her home, if that is not the patient's wish it will not succeed and alternative resources will always be needed as was demonstrated by an elderly gentleman. He had insisted he wanted to go into residential care but, although fairly frail, his medical condition cleared and the consultant insisted on his discharge. Once home, Bill sat in his chair unable to move, incontinent and miserable. An emergency place was found in a residential home and, when the social worker went to collect him, he got out of his chair, put on his cap and walked to the door!

A small but growing group of people who come to the social worker's attention are the couples where one requires nursing and the other residential care and who may be separated without any consideration for their emotional needs. They may perhaps spend the last years of their lives apart because no one has realised they would wish to be together. It is only if they have extensive financial resources that they can move into a dual registered private nursing home. However, it is worth discussing the situation further with local authorities since if one member, even the bedfast one, is the 'brains' and the other, even if confused, is the 'legs' of the partnership it may be possible that they can enter a local authority elderly persons' home together. It is always worth remembering that a couple may not necessarily be husband and wife but any two people who have spent most of their adult years together.

9.5   *The confused elderly person*

This section deals with confusion as encountered on a general hospital ward and not dementia. The condition even in a mild form often provokes a protectiveness from nursing staff which could cause the social worker to doubt the wisdom of a return home; however it should be remembered that once in familiar surroundings the confusion can lessen and the answer is not to arrange Part III to keep the person safe unless all other options have been explored.

As with any other elderly person, it is the person's right to be consulted and it is courteous to check if she minds before contacting a relative.

All clients particularly those with dementia have the right to be informed. The right to be informed about plans for the future, treatment received, risks run and more controversially about their diagnosis. They have the right to be upset: they have the right to be listened to and believed.[5]

Probably the most difficult area in working with the confused person is having any sort of meaningful communication. It takes time and patience and preferably interviews should be conducted privately, thus lessening the embarrassment the social worker may feel with the eyes of the ward fixed on her and hearing comments like 'she won't remember anything'. It is vital to remember to face the person to get eye contact if possible and

to speak in short sentences using simple words and not to ask
long and convoluted questions. However:

The secret to successful communication lies not so much in the learning
of particular techniques but in each worker believing implicitly in the
worth of the confused person and the need to talk with them, involve
them in decisions and take account of their preferences.[6]

Some confused people will confabulate and this can catch the
unwary or inexperienced social worker out as was demonstrated
by one old gentleman. He convinced the worker that he was
coping well at home, doing his own cooking and shopping and
was completely unsupported by family or friends. She suggested
to the ward sister that a time of convalescence might be helpful
as he had to go home to do his own work and was living alone.
At which point the ward sister roared with laughter and asked
where he would go. Apparently he got dressed every evening
and stood in the middle of the upstairs ward waiting for his
bus to take him home from the pub! He thought the ward
was the 'local' and on checking with his family it was further
discovered that the degree of help afforded to him by his son
and family was extremely high. During the follow up visits to
his home the degree of his confusion became more evident.

It may be that there is concern about the client's ability to
manage her own affairs. Figure 9.1 is produced from a Kings
Fund Project Paper.[7] The document is a useful guide to both
Court of Protection and guardianship and it is the latter power
which a hospital social worker may need to invoke with a very
confused elderly person if it is felt necessary to admit her to an
elderly persons' home for her own safety and she is refusing,
or can't make the decision to go. It is worth noting however
that although the Act gives the guardian the right to decide
where the person shall live, it does not give the guardian the
right to remove the person forcefully from the hospital bed!

9.6   Elderly people from ethnic minority groups

A game called 'Ba-fa-ba' is sometimes used on training courses.
Course members are divided into two teams and each is given
its own rules.

Is the client mentally disordered?

YES ←——　——→ NO

NO branch:

2b. Is there concern that he or she may become mentally disturbed?

– NO – Then no action seems necessary though the client may wish to create an ordinary general power of attorney.

YES

YES branch:

2a. Is he or she nevertheless still able to manage his or her property and affairs?

– YES – Then he or she can do so but it could still be wise to investigate his or her ability to make an enduring power of attorney.

NO

3a. Is he or she about to act in a way that will leave him or her with less money or property?

– YES – Consider (a) applying for an emergency order from the Court of Protection, and (b) advising the other party that the client is mentally disordered so that the gift or contract may be invalid.

3b. Does he or she want to agree to having his or her property and finances reorganised so that he or she is likely to be able to manage even if mentally disordered?

– YES – Then make such arrangements But also consider 4b.

NO

4a. Does he or she obtain a civil service or military pension?

– YES – Then ask the Paymaster General or Ministry of Defence to make it payable to someone else.

NO

4b. Does the client or someone else wish to create a trust for a trustee to administer and 'own' the property?

– YES – Then make such arrangements but note that trust property often still belongs to the people it benefits when calculating their

5a. Does he or she obtain any social security?

– YES – Then approach the local DSS to have an appointee appointed.

NO

5b. Does he or she wish to appoint someone to look after his or her property should he or she become mentally disordered?

– YES – Then he or she should make an enduring power of attorney being careful to specify what he or she wants done.

NO

charges for Part III accommodation and supplementary benefit.

6a. Are the client's finances and property relatively easy to collect together and administer and around £5,000 or less?

– YES – Then consider applying to the CoP for a short procedure order.

NO

6b. Then no action is appropriate although the client should be warned that if he or she becomes mentally disordered then any ordinary power of attorney will be invalid and an expensive application to the CoP may be necessary.

NO

Consider applying to the CoP for a receivership order. Note the medical and legal tests.

Figure 9.1. Bringing in the Court of Protection.

The object is to find out what rules govern the behaviour of the other team whilst having no previous knowledge of them. It is surprisingly difficult and frustrating particularly as each team is also given a new vocabulary. For some of the elderly people from the ethnic minority groups living in this country it must be rather like playing that game. As they become older and their families move away and relatives and friends are dying, the elderly person becomes isolated and health breaks down and an admission to hospital must be a very frightening event.

The culture of the hospital can be totally alien to someone who can understand what is being said and what is happening but, for an elderly person who has always been protected and never learned the language and customs of this country, the experience will be extremely frightening and bewildering. Equally, there may be a lack of understanding of religious and cultural customs among hospital staff making that person feel even more isolated. For the social worker there may be even greater pressure than usual about the discharge because of lack of appropriate resources and it may be useful to employ a professional interpreter rather than a family member in order to understand the true position and wishes of the person. The social worker may also be able to help in educating ward staff and, particularly in an area where there are only small numbers of people from ethnic minority groups, may be able to pick up racist attitudes or insensitivity to cultural issues. Conflicts can arise about food and the custom of bringing all the food into the ward may cause problems initially. Likewise the custom of immediate burial posed one hospital a problem as a body could not be released to the waiting relatives. Perhaps the area where most sensitivity is needed is the use now made of mixed wards and the difficulty this can cause to a lady who practises purdah.

9.7   *People with a sensory handicap*

The deaf or blind person on the hospital ward may have a similar experience of isolation. Boredom can be a particular problem. A social worker was able to arrange for talking books and a tape recorder to be loaned to a blind lady who had been on the ward for some months and for the deaf person a deaf signer volunteer may help to alleviate some of the problems.

A group for profoundly deaf long-stay patients may be an appropriate vehicle for alleviating isolation. If residential care is needed there are elderly persons' homes specifically for people with these handicaps.

9.8   The social worker and the supervisor

Much has been said about the rights, needs and wishes of the elderly person and the carers, little mention has so far been made of the social worker's needs. Work with elderly persons takes a considerable degree of patience, insight, knowledge and creativity and, as has been demonstrated, family work is often of paramount importance. The degree of anxiety experienced by the social worker, medical and nursing staff when the elderly, very frail person returns home against everyone's advice may be acute and the frustration at lack of resources inevitably takes a great deal of the social worker's emotional energy.

The supervisor will need to recognise these pressures and to support the worker's decision to respect the client's wishes. It was commented by a social worker that she felt isolated and alone in coordinating plans for a discharge and that other disciplines within the hospital, whom she would have expected to help implement those plans, seemed to block every suggestion made. This resulted in the social worker feeling she was in a no-win situation, being pressurised by the consultants to clear the bed and listening to nursing staff and family begging her to find a safe place, and the patient's wishes to go home. It was necessary for the supervisor and social worker to talk through the client's rights and wishes, the relatives' rights and wishes and the overt and covert agendas of the other disciplines before an objective view could be obtained and maintained. In these situations it is easy for the social worker to become the scapegoat for consultants and other doctors because of pressure on beds and lack of appropriate NHS resources, and for the nursing staff because they cannot be sure the community will be able to provide the necessary care. The social worker may well need help to decide what is her responsibility, what she can do something about, what she can change and what the other disciplines within the hospital must take on as their own responsibility.

Both the social worker and supervisor need to be in touch with their feelings about their own ageing process and that of their relatives. Many workers will have elderly parents themselves and since a high proportion of hospital social workers are women it is likely they are involved in the care of a widowed mother or father. It may well be that before she can work objectively with elderly people she will have to look at her own role and relationships within her family and to realise that professional objectivity should not be confused with being a caring daughter. While the latter may give insight and empathy into a client's family situation, to identify too deeply with any one member could lead to sympathy and collusion and the view of the case could become muddled and biased to the detriment of the client.

Ageing is an experience that is common to everyone, cannot be denied or hidden from, is inevitable and implacable, and the worker must value what she is doing and accept the elements of risk-taking in order to help her elderly client achieve the most desirable quality of life possible given her present life situation and health.

No chapter can give an exhaustive list of all the issues that need to be considered or that are likely to be present in working with this client group. Some issues such as counselling for bereavement and loss are universal and are dealt with elsewhere in the book. The aim of this chapter has been to raise awareness and consciousness of some of the common areas that occur when working with the elderly person but most importantly to bring out the value of this work at a time when there is often impatience and scant respect for age. The following (anonymous) poem states these issues clearly.

> What do you see, nurses, what do you see?
> What are you thinking when you are looking at me?
> A crabbit old woman not very wise,
> Uncertain of habit with far-away eyes,
> Who dribbles her food and makes no reply
> When you say in a loud voice 'I do wish you'd try',
> Who seems not to notice the things that you do,
> And forever is losing a stocking or shoe,
> Who unresisting or not lets you do as you will,

With bathing and feeding the long day to fill,
Is that what you are thinking, is that what you see?
Then open your eyes, nurse, you are not looking at me.
I'll tell you who I am as I sit here so still,
As I rise at your bidding as I eat at your will.
I'm a small child of ten with a father and mother,
Brothers and sisters who love one another,
A young girl of sixteen with wings on her feet
Dreaming that soon now a lover she'll meet,
A bride soon at twenty my heart gives a leap,
Remembering the vows that I promised to keep,
At twenty-five now I have young of my own
Who need me to build a secure, happy home,
A woman of thirty my young now grow fast
Bound to each other with ties that should last,
At forty my young sons now grow and will be gone
But my man stays beside me to see I don't mourn,
At fifty once more babes play round my knee,
Again we know children, my loved ones and me.
Dark days are upon me, my husband is dead,
I look at the future, I shudder with dread,
For my young are all busy rearing young of their own
And I think of the years and the love that I've known.
I'm an old woman now and nature is cruel,'
'Tis her jest to make old age look like a fool.
The body it crumbles, grace and vigour depart,
There is now a stone where I once had a heart,
But inside this carcase where a young girl still dwells
And now and again my battered heart swells,
I remember the joys, I remember the pain,
And I'm loving and living life all over again.
I think of the years all too few – gone too fast
And accept the stark fact that nothing can last,
So open your eyes, nurse, open and see
Not a crabbit old woman, look closer –

see ME!

Notes

1. Redding, D., 'Age discrimination: Problematic term', *Community Care*, 25 May 1989.
2. National Assistance Act 1948, Part III.

3. Norman, Alison J., *'Right and Risks': A discussion document on civil liberty in old age,* published by NCCOP, 1980, p. 18.
4. Information made available by Age Concern.
5. Good, Val, 'Speak listen learn and help,' *Social Work Today,* 4 May 1989.
6. *ibid.*
7. Carson, David (ed.), *Making the Most of the Court of Protection,* Kings Fund, 1987.

Suggestions for further reading

De Beauvoir, Simone, *Old Age,* Harmondsworth: Penguin, 1970.

Discharge of Patients from Hospital, DHSS Health Circular HC (89)5; Local Authority Circular LAC (89)7, Crown Copyright, February 1989.

Griffiths, Sir Roy, *Community Care: Agenda for action,* report to the Secretary of State for social services, HMSO: London, 1988.

Marris, Peter, *Loss and Change,* London: Routledge & Kegan Paul, 1989.

Marshall, Mary, *Social Work with old people,* BASW Practical Social Work series, (ed.) Jo Campling, Macmillan Education, 1989.

CHAPTER 10

Conclusion

MIEKE BADAWI and BRENDA BIAMONTI

The *raison d'etre* of the hospital-based social worker is in helping people to cope with the social and emotional effects of acute or chronic illness and disability. This contribution to health care is essential to maintaining a view of the patient as a whole person, with an entire life that is being affected by the present illness and hospitalisation. This has been discussed from a variety of perspectives throughout the preceding pages and we hope it has made a useful contribution to the literature on social work in health care. We have echoed Sofia Butrym's themes, expanded on them and given them a practice oriented expression. Butrym says:

The central characteristic of medical social work is its direct concern with the social and emotional problems connected with illness and its medical treatment, and with any consequent adjustments in the lives of patients and their families. It follows from this that constant encounters with the problem of physical pain, mental anguish, various forms of mutilation, and death, are a major feature of the work . . . . The ability to sense and respond appropriately to [these feelings of] apprehension and fear is an essential qualification for being able to help such people. This requires both an appreciation of the needs of this group to which both psychological and sociological knowledge offer an important contribution, and also a certain type of personality and a degree of maturity to enable the worker to contain the emotional stress inherent in trying to meet these particular needs. For a medical social worker a degree of success in coming to terms herself with the unavoidability of death and a capacity to tolerate both physical pain and depression, are quite indispensable.[1]

191

There are certain themes within this book, which are mentioned by almost all our contributors.

Bereavement counselling and grief work which account for a very large proportion of time in all hospital social work specialisms. This is seen as a cornerstone of the social worker's task by all contributors. The practical work social workers undertake on behalf of their clients, and which is seen by some colleagues, both in social work and in other professions as their only duty, is felt to be a beginning. Practical social work tasks, efficiently fulfilled are part of any social worker's job. They are also an essential first step which helps the worker gain the trust of the client and may, most hospital social workers hope, lead to what some see as their most important one, namely counselling. However, it is interesting that many contributors have stressed how important it is to be 'reliably alongside', to have 'respect for persons' and not to force counselling upon anyone. Whether her counselling skills are called upon or not, the worker will need to have a sound understanding of the grieving processes involved, both within her clients and within herself.

Recent times have seen a particular interest in approaches to treatment for and care of the dying. A fresh impetus has been given to this preoccupation by the increase of untimely deaths from AIDS. We have not treated this as a separate subject partly because the skills that are employed in helping and counselling are the same ones that hospital social workers can be called upon to employ any day in working with people, very often young people who are dying.

Effective co-operation with colleagues from other professional groups and being optimally effective in a field, health, that is dominated by the medical profession is still a preoccupation for all our contributors, as it has been since medical social work began. (See especially Chapters 1, 3 and 9.) This aspect of the work has been the subject of much debate within the field. The word co-operation confirms for some images of 'the handmaiden' or the pseudo-medic in the white coat. Paul Bywaters makes the point forcefully when he suggests a 'social model of health for social work practice'.[2] He goes on to argue:

The roles played by social workers in hospitals are largely determined by members of other occupational groups and social workers frequently find themselves attempting to work in situations unsympathetic to their own perceptions of the needs of their clients/patients. They are exhorted in the literature of social work to act as partners, when many experience their position as being barely tolerated visitors.

He also reminds us that health is not the sole province of medicine and that generally speaking doctors concern themselves with *ill* health and treatment by medical means, whereas social workers are concerned with what maintains *good* health. They try to help create conditions that may prevent the forerunners of ill health: physical, social and emotional stress, or to minimise the ill-effects of 'the slings and arrows of outrageous fortune'.

Advocacy is a strong linking theme through the book. Several of our authors have written of the necessity to separate themselves, psychologically at least, from the institution if they are to keep a person/client orientation. They know well the effects of institutionalisation on both themselves (and indeed on other professionals who work within the NHS) and clients (see Chapters 5, 7 and 9). Advocacy, on the client's behalf is immensely important within and without the hospital, with other hospital staff, with families and with outside agencies (Chapters 2, 6, 8 and 9). It is therefore necessary for the workers not to become institutionalised and take on wholesale the values of their workplace.

Work in area-based social work departments can have different perspectives and priorities from work within a hospital social work department. For this reason difficulties can arise when there is a gap between the hospital-based social worker's assessment of need and what an area social work department sees as important or is able to provide. It may therefore become necessary to press for the provision of certain services.

We have also been told in the preceding pages about the *stress factor*, the 'there but for the Grace of God' feeling that assails hospital social workers quite frequently. Working with sick, suffering human beings day in, day out, working with the elderly and/or the chronically sick, where there is no improvement expected, indeed where there is only a downward slope in prospect, can have a depressing effect on the social worker. To help them cope they need good support from colleagues, regular, supportive and frequent supervision, and ideally some time out when things are getting really rough (Chapters 4, 5, and

9). Many managers feel that they need mature and experienced workers in the hospitals. But, however mature and experienced the worker may be, we do not think we could stress strongly enough how important first-class supervision and support is. Only a well-supported social worker can give well-planned and thought-out help to her clients.

The isolation and specialisation, which are typical of the way hospital social work tends to be organised (see below and Chapters 2, 3 and 5), also mean that stress and distress are difficult to share and diffuse if supervision is not forthcoming. There is some debate about how this can best be achieved. On the one hand there is the view that the social work manager/supervisor should be a practitioner herself in order to keep in touch with practice so as to understand fully the current stresses endured. On the other hand there is the view that the manager/supervisor must be available for staff support and consultation at all times. This part of the argument states that a manager's first priority and loyalty should be to the staff. If she also has a case-load, a conflict of interest might arise.

Stress and social worker burnout can be caused by the strain of working closely with people who have different sets of values (see above) and holding on to her self-confidence, and confidence in the value of the work she is doing. In some hospitals there is a long tradition of social work, and the majority of the staff are aware of the social worker's contribution, but even here there are always staff changes, new and/or young recruits have to be taught from scratch. In other hospitals there is little or no tradition, or the expectations of the institution (Chapter 1) have been allowed to take precedence and the wrong kind of tradition has developed. The worker has to be very sure of herself not to be unduly influenced by the prevailing climate of opinion amongst those with whom she works daily and to stick to her own and her department's standards and priorities.

Work with people with a different cultural background has been approached mainly in Chapter 7 (but see also Chapter 9), an indication perhaps how right the author is in pointing out that not enough attention is paid to this very important subject in Britain in 1990. The chapter exposes weaknesses in anti-racist training of social workers, and in their practice in working with people from ethnic minorities. The author uses 'racist' as a term to cover both colour prejudice and lack of sensitivity to and understanding of different cultures. 'Black' is used to describe anyone who is not 'white'. These are usages which may strike some people as confusing, but which seem to have become accepted by many people writing on these issues. Racism and the undervaluing of anyone seen as different is rife and blatant in our society and must be fought against by all of us. People with disabilities face a similar prejudice: the wheelchair, the lack of sight, like the skin-colour, is the first thing – perhaps even the only thing – that is noticed about people and they are treated and approached in a stereotyped manner, the disabled person as if she were lacking in all senses, and the black person according to the interlocutor's preconceived ideas about her race and/or culture.

The degree of *specialisation* that exists within hospital social work has perhaps not been sufficiently stressed, although it may have become obvious in the examples chosen for some chapters. Social workers do their work in isolation, as individuals. They tend to work in units (Chapter 3), which, besides its obvious advantages for the worker, in that she accumulates a great deal of specialised knowledge, and has great freedom of action, has grave disadvantages. In some units, specially those dealing with chronic illness, where there is a strong 'unit culture', adhered to by staff and patients alike, it becomes almost impossible for the social worker not to identify too strongly with this culture, and to maintain the necessary distance. There is a difficulty here: on the one hand, it makes for better working relationships if the social worker becomes very much part of the team in the institution, and patients will feel this as a positive thing too. However, there is the fact that the social worker belongs to a different bureaucracy, and that her management may well have different priorities from those of NHS management (Chapter 2).

Another disadvantage is that the specialised knowledge accumulated may become 'private knowledge', and is often not shared; it can lead to empire building: the worker talks about 'my wards, my team' and may become jealous about allowing other social workers on 'her patch'. It may suit the individualist, but is probably not healthy for the overall practice of social work in hospitals. Being so private/secretive is wasteful of expertise above all else.

We have tried to share some of our knowledge, but for reasons of space and readability we were not able to cover all aspects of social work in hospitals. We hope that this book will act as a stimulus for other colleagues to write about their own private knowledge and experience. The chest clinic social worker might tell us about the fact that there one meets more people of 'no fixed abode' than almost anywhere else; if you sleep rough you are likely to get recurrent chest-infections or chronic bronchitis. In plastic surgery the worker might become a specialist in helping people with gender difficulties: it is there where they get help in changing their bodies to suit their feelings about themselves. General medicine treats countless different conditions, like disorders (physical and/or psychological) where people become so obese that they need hospital treatment, like the 40-odd-year-old bachelor who said he was 'married to his frying pan'. Rheumatology may introduce us to carers who are 'willing victims', but where patients get to know their disease very well indeed, like the old man, who said: 'There is nothing like despondency to knock your health about, is there?'

Hospital social work is a crossroads at present. The White Paper on the reorganisation of the NHS, *Working for Patients* does not address the implications for social work services, while the implications of the more recent White Paper on community care, *Caring for People*, are vast (see Chapter 2). Planning discharges to the community of disabled and/or elderly people will become an ever-increasing part of the social workers' duties. As people live longer, and survive disabling illness, or are medically enabled to live and to be discharged to the community with chronic illnesses that used to kill and 'new' diseases are diagnosed and treated, hospitals and their ability to give complete treatment to the whole person are, and always will be, an important part of any civilised society. May social workers continue to play their part in keeping our society civilised!

Notes

1. Butrym, Sofia, *The Nature of Medical Social Work*, London: Routledge & Kegan Paul, 1967.
2. Bywaters, Paul, 'Social work and the medical profession: Arguments against unconditional collaboration', *British Journal of Social Work*, **16**, 1986, pp. 661–77.

Index

197